616.0472 F5331p 2014
Fisher, Keren, author
The practical pain
management handbook : the
essential evidence-based
guide
34

The Practical Pain Management Handbook

THE ESSENTIAL EVIDENCE-BASED GUIDE

D0162871

DR KEREN FISHER
Clinical Psychologist

and

DR SUSAN CHILDS
Clinical Psychologist

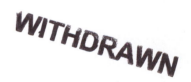

Forewords by

PROFESSOR LANCE McCRACKEN
Professor of Behavioural Medicine
King's College London

and

DR GLYN TOWLERTON
BSc MRCP FRCA FIPP FFPMRCA
Consultant in Pain Medicine

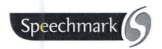
Speechmark

CUYAHOGA COMMUNITY COLLEGE
EASTERN CAMPUS LIBRARY

First published in 2014 by
Speechmark Publishing Ltd, St Mark's House, Shepherdess Walk,
London N1 7BQ, UK
Tel: +44 (0)20 7954 3400

www.speechmark.net

© Keren Fisher and Susan Childs, 2014

All rights reserved. The whole of this work, including all text and illustrations, is protected by copyright. No part of it may be copied, altered, adapted or otherwise exploited in any way without express prior permission, unless in accordance with the provisions of the Copyright Designs and Patents Act 1988 or in order to photocopy or make duplicating masters of those pages so indicated, without alteration and including copyright notices, for the express purpose of instruction and examination. No parts of this work may otherwise be loaded, stored, manipulated, reproduced, or transmitted in any form or by any means, electronic or mechanical, including photocopying and recording, or by any information storage and retrieval system, without prior written permission from the publisher, on behalf of the copyright owner.

002-5963/Printed in the United Kingdom by CMP (uk) Ltd
Designed and typeset by Darkriver Design, Auckland, New Zealand
British Library Cataloguing in Publication Data
A catalogue record for this book is available from the British Library

ISBN 978 190930 109 2

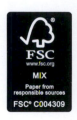

Contents

CONTENTS

Foreword by Professor Lance McCracken

PRACTICAL HELP FOR THOSE WITH PAIN AND ALL THOSE WHO SUPPORT THEM

The problem of persistent pain imposes a huge burden on us humans. When it is present it can take control and impose its agenda. It can discourage, intimidate and frighten, not only the person directly suffering with pain, but their loved ones, and even those professionals who they seek for help. Of course, for the intended audience of this book, these experiences are well known. It almost appears repetitious or even gloomy to describe them yet again. At the same time, they are a starting point – these words are to say 'we are in this together'. Whichever stake you claim here, patient, family, friend or treatment provider, the authors of this book are here to join you, to reach out a hand and help.

It may surprise some to learn that, in this day of ultra-high tech medical diagnostics and treatments, chronic pain remains uncontrolled for a large proportion of the world's population. In fact with all of our advances in medical technology and knowledge of pain today, the results many people experience in treatment are very similar to results achieved more than 20 years ago, no worse but no better either. Still, there are rays of hope. Today, 14 years into the 21st century, some of the brightest rays of hope emerge from within current psychological approaches to chronic pain, specifically those referred to broadly as 'cognitive behavioural therapy' or CBT. If we look to such resources as the authoritative Cochrane Library of reviews (www.thecochranelibrary.com), we see that these approaches have a large evidence base – we know they help. They can change how people experience their pain, how distressed they feel, and what they are able to do about it. Unlike medical approaches to chronic pain, the power of these approaches comes not from 'high technology' methods that can be done for you or to you, but from things each of us can do for ourselves. The real power of these approaches resides in the remarkable fact of human potential, the ability to learn, to change our behaviour or to persist, to meet adversity and keep moving, in one way or another. Each of us is remarkably able to lose our way, to find it again and to follow 'our way', particularly if we are provided help when we feel most stuck and downhearted. Here 'our way' means our hopes and dreams, our plans in life and our goals. So that there will be no misunderstanding, there is 'high technology' here. It is simply not pharmacology, chemistry or biology, but the technology of human interaction and behaviour change.

For those who experience chronic pain the range of methods for responding to it has developed and expanded significantly during recent years, as this practical handbook clearly shows. Now there are methods we might call standard cognitive behavioural, mindfulness-based, and others we can call acceptance and commitment therapy, or ACT. With this expansion there are now more options for the chronic pain stakeholders. This means that people with chronic pain can learn about these options and choose where to begin. Also, if one set of methods does not prove successful, another set can be used, provided that enough help and supports can be found in each of these cases.

So, what about the future, how will each of us stay fresh, effective and up-to-date in our learning and skills? No current psychological treatment approach for any problem has achieved the status as the perfect treatment, or the 'last word' in treatment development, and no approach is yet 100% effective. Overall, some of the treatment methods used today are different from those used 20 years ago, and 20 years from now they are certain to be, once again, different from today. For one thing, we know that packages of treatments that include the method outlined here can produce real benefits for people. This is not the same, however, as saying that all of the methods here will create equal benefit for all people. Substantial, equal and lasting benefits for all people remain objectives to reach.

Many of the methods included in the handbook probably operate on the same few processes of change. This is good news! This means that for each of the primary challenges chronic pain holds for a person there are several ways to address that challenge, and it is possible to experiment to see which ones fit best and achieve the best results. One day, researchers and treatment providers will identify these key challenges and key processes of change. They will also find ways to deliver treatments so that they are sensitive to individuals' particular treatment needs, so that they are customised and tailored to fit. And finally, they will help us to achieve health care delivery systems where all pain management services are uniformly skilful and high quality for all who need them. If we can master these three aims, processes of change, matching treatments to needs and high-quality delivery, then the burden of chronic pain is likely to be much lighter than it is today, one day.

So, in the meantime, it is time to begin. If you are reading this book so far, it must mean that there are goals you want to achieve *and* you are not achieving them. If these goals are important enough to you, perhaps you will take the next step. Read on. And remember, although you will at times feel alone, you are not alone.

Lance M McCracken, PhD
Professor of Behavioural Medicine
King's College London
June 2014

Foreword by Dr Glyn Towlerton

This is an excellent self-help book for helpers to help support self-help in others. Many people espouse the benefits of a structured pain management programme without really understanding the nuts and bolts this entails. Within these pages I hope you will find an excellent dissection of therapies to help patients.

To distil nearly 40 years of hard-won expertise and experience into a clear concise manual is an achievement which should be recognised. This is not a book to discuss the evidence bases around delivery of care but filters the provision of care as specific isolated packages of help in a clear and concise manner. It may in part help unify different groups' approaches to pain management and explore the best contemporary knowledge to the benefit of those dealing with the chronic pain population, which is of course much larger than we like to acknowledge. Even those not directly involved in the provision of pain management programmes but involved in any patient in pain's care would benefit from the knowledge in these pages. The best teams function by knowing a little of what each member is trying to deliver and I would commend this to all those involved in treating pain patients for their day-to-day practice but also understanding of what is and what is not possible in behavioural modification.

We often say that the pain does not go away, just the pain patient does. At least with the knowledge herein you may hope that if the patient does leave, at least it will be with the tools to enable them to tackle this most insidious symptom and improve their quality of life.

Dr Glyn Towlerton
BSc MRCP FRCA FIPP FFPMRCA
Consultant in Pain Medicine
June 2014

About the authors

Dr Keren Fisher qualified as a clinical psychologist in the 1970s and gained a PhD through researching the emotional and cognitive factors that influence the relationship between disability and chronic pain. She instituted pain management programmes in the Royal National Orthopaedic Hospital in London and has been developing psychological theories in the delivery of pain management for more than 30 years. Her specialist interest is currently in clinical and research activities with people with post-amputation (phantom limb) pain.

Dr Susan Childs is a consultant clinical psychologist with the Chelsea and Westminster Hospital NHS Foundation Trust in the Pain Management Service. She has specialised in chronic pain since her doctorate in 1999 and has written and provided both one-to-one and group services for a number of trusts. She has written and developed the service specification for five differing pain management groups to meet the wide spectrum of need in this specific population and has instigated dual services aimed at meeting the needs of patients with psychosocial, psychiatric or unusual pain presentation issues. Her main therapeutic model is cognitive behavioural therapy but she has developed the use of acceptance and commitment therapy and mindfulness models within group and one-to-one interventions. She sees this book as an amalgamation of practice, experience and thinking from her last 20 years of practice.

Introduction for Therapists

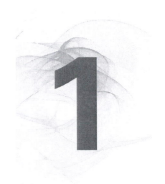

The successful management of chronic pain remains an elusive goal. As more complex diagnostic and intervention procedures become available, patients and clinicians alike have ever-greater expectations of banishing the problem of pain altogether. Unfortunately this hope is rarely fulfilled and the frustration experienced by everyone affected by chronic pain has remained more or less the same over the last two or three decades.

Pain management programmes (PMPs) are popular for their ability to help patients and their families understand and cope with the transmission of abnormal neural stimulation, its subsequent experience as pain and its related disability, distress and adverse life effects. However, programmes vary in their mode of delivery and in their inputs and outcomes. There is no absolute format, as each programme will depend on the available resources and current thinking.

For many years we have been using and adapting mental health texts to meet the needs of our chronic pain patients. It struck us that there should be a book specifically for therapists involved in running PMPs and we recognised the need to have access to a greater variety of suitable teaching and interactive materials than we could find.

Between us we have over 40 years' experience of learning from our mistakes and trying to hone our programmes until they are as engaging and effective as possible. The information in this handbook is the result of our most developed thoughts and accumulated know-how to date, but of course there will always be new ideas, political interests and research findings to change the prevailing philosophy.

We have discovered that there are both gains and losses to be had from both intensive inpatient and extended outpatient programmes, as long as they are of at least 25 hours in length, with about 8–12 patients in a group. Smaller numbers dilute the social learning effect and may reduce the cost-effectiveness of the programme. Shorter programmes are reported to be less effective.

Whether you choose to have inpatient or outpatient programmes depends on your resources. The British Pain Society reports that the degree of patients' distress and disability may contribute more to treatment outcomes than whether or not the patients are residential. The core recommendation is that the staff should be specifically experienced and involve (in addition to a medically qualified person) a chartered clinical or health psychologist (or a suitably qualified cognitive behavioural therapist) and a chartered physiotherapist. The addition of a nurse and occupational therapist with specific competencies in chronic pain management is a great advantage.

We suggest the programme format needs to begin with a multidisciplinary assessment session. While this might involve patients still having to wait for admission to the main bulk of the programme, information is discussed during the assessment that enables patients to understand the principles they will encounter in later weeks and which significantly reduces the drop-out rate once the programme has started. We discovered the assessment session began the process of change, so patients joined the programme already experiencing less pain and distress than had been identified at referral.

We also found that follow-up sessions (which could occur incrementally at three months, six months and a year) in which important outcome data should be recorded, were not often well attended. To address this common problem we began encouraging patients to attend by offering them a variety of booster workshops in which they could revise their skills in stretching exercises, relaxation and mindfulness, cognitive challenges, problem solving or new goal attainment. These workshops have proved to be enjoyable and successful.

We have organised this handbook into the sections we think fit a useful logical sequence but you must adapt them to suit your preference. Some sections require more than one session. You must split up the material as you think fit.

The material really needs to form the basis of group discussion rather than didactic teaching. Where there is a question in the text the suggested answer material is provided, but you may wish to withhold this while you ask for contributing answers from the participants. In our experience we find that the most important messages are best remembered through the language the patients generate themselves.

Where assignments are given as homework, ask for feedback and reports of any problems at the beginning of the very next session. When we inadvertently forgot to do this ourselves, we found compliance dropped off and learning opportunities were missed.

We have incorporated both standard cognitive behavioural therapy (CBT) and acceptance and commitment therapy (ACT) technologies, as both have been found to be valuable in PMPs. The table presented in this introduction shows the similarities and differences between CBT and ACT techniques, which may be of use to you in planning your sessions.

While we generally believe the mindfulness approach to defusing the influence of thoughts on actions is valuable, our experience has shown that particularly persistent or 'sticky' thoughts benefit more from a CBT approach.

Pages headed 'A task for you' can be homework or group session exercises. Therapists involved in running PMPs should refer to the enclosed CD for printable versions of the Tasks. However, Section 18 (Pain Management Programme Problem Pages) is intended to

Speechmark ☺ ⓟ This page may be photocopied for instructional use only © 2014 Keren Fisher and Susan Childs

be a group assignment – we suggest you copy the pages and cut them up into separate problems so patients can choose which ones they would like to work on.

DIFFERENCES BETWEEN TRADITIONAL COGNITIVE BEHAVIOURAL THERAPY AND ACCEPTANCE AND COMMITMENT THERAPY

CBT encourages people to analyse their thought content and to see how it has influenced their emotions and reactions.

ACT, on the other hand, asks people to reduce the influence of thoughts on emotions and actions and to see thoughts as just passing events in the mind. Thoughts don't need to be glued or fused to a particular response. Instead, ACT encourages *action guided by life values.*

Principal CBT techniques	Principal ACT techniques
Encourages detailed examination of thoughts (Exactly what were the thoughts in that situation?)	Attempts to remove influence of thoughts on emotion and behaviour
Analyses thoughts for 'distortions' or 'errors'	Encourages thoughts to pass along as events in the mind without judging them
Looks for alternative thoughts or interpretations of a situation	Uses metaphors to encourage new views of a situation (e.g. if in a hole, trying to dig a way out will aggravate the situation)
Uses verbal questions to clarify 'meaning' of thoughts or interpretations of a situation	Discourages analysing thoughts for meaning
Looks for evidence to prove or disprove thoughts	Reduces emphasis on verbal 'rules'
Seeks to change verbal interpretation in view of evidence	Encourages discovery of what is helpful via experience
Keeps its focus on verbal influence of thoughts on emotion and behaviour	Keeps its focus on awareness of present moment-to-moment experience
Focuses on moving towards tangible goals	Focuses on moving in the direction of life values
Uses Behavioural experiments	Uses Behavioural experiments
Uses Homework tasks	Uses Homework tasks

We would appreciate feedback from your experience of running programmes based on this handbook. We can be contacted via Speechmark Publishing Ltd.

Dr Keren Fisher
Consultant Clinical Psychologist
Dr Susan Childs
Consultant Clinical Psychologist
June 2014

Speechmark Ⓟ This page may be photocopied for instructional use only © 2014 Keren Fisher and Susan Childs

Pain Management Programme Introduction: Multidisciplinary Assessment Session

This session is about assessing how your pain affects your life and how you are dealing with it. You will have a chance to learn more about the pain management programme you have been referred for. Pain management programmes are *not about curing pain* (we don't know enough to be able to offer you this) but you will have a chance to learn about understanding chronic (long-term) pain and the things you can do to reduce its impact on your life.

In this assessment session, we can help you begin to learn the basic messages about pain. There may be some questionnaires to fill in about how you feel and how the pain problem affects your thoughts and beliefs, emotions and behaviours. You may be asked to take part in a few activities to see how you get on.

The main message that forms the basis of changing the effects of pain is that

> pain is produced by the brain, but this is not to say it's all in the mind, imaginary, psychosomatic or unreal.

The mind and the brain are not the same. The brain receives information from stimulation in the nervous system and the mind influences how the brain responds by adding thoughts, beliefs, memories and emotions in the form of more nerve impulses. The brain acts as the control centre that adds all the information together and produces a pain response. So, the more sources of stimulation the brain receives, the more information is added to the experience of pain.

Even *acute pain*, usually related to tissue damage like a sprain or fracture, is produced by the brain. The main function of the brain is to keep you alive and warn you of danger. A person with a new injury will be in pain because the brain creates danger messages. The patient takes whatever treatment steps are appropriate to restore the damaged tissue to full health and the brain turns off the danger signals.

However, once the pain has persisted beyond the 3–6 months it takes for the tissues to heal, the brain is no longer responding to injury in the body but to the *increased sensitivity*

Speechmark ☉ ℗ This page may be photocopied for instructional use only © 2014 Keren Fisher and Susan Childs *of the nervous system*, which has developed over the months the danger signals have been firing. There are now complex messages flowing to and from the brain about the biological, psychological and social environment that affect the nerve impulses. The brain is stuck in danger mode, so the *treatment now has to focus on training the brain to wind down* the sensitivity of the nervous system.

Chronic or long-term pain now looks like Figure 1. All the secondary causes are nerve impulses too, which all add to the brain's danger response. Brain training starts with reducing the effects of these problems.

TAKING THE BROAD VIEW OF LONG-TERM PAIN

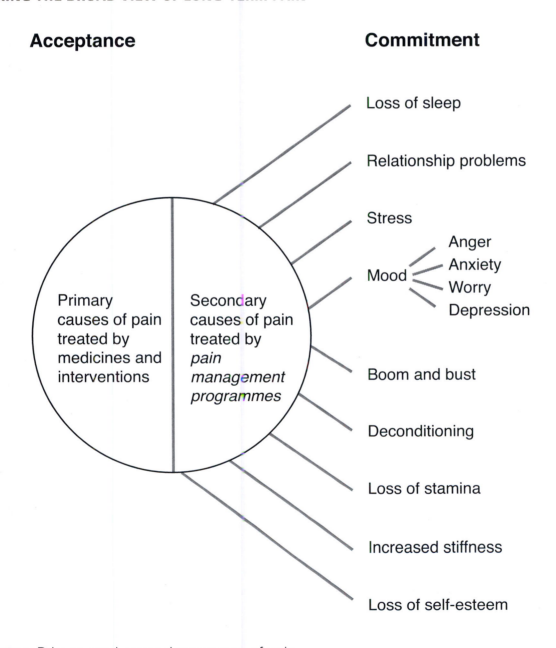

FIGURE 1 Primary and secondary causes of pain

Speechmark P This page may be photocopied for instructional use only © 2014 Keren Fisher and Susan Childs

STRUCTURE OF THE PROGRAMME

There will be sessions dealing with all the factors that influence your pain, your mood and their impact on your life.

You will be able to learn better techniques for improving sleep, stress and pain-related problems in your relationships. Most important, you will have a chance to consider what is really important in your life – your values, and you will learn how to work on goal activities related to them. This will involve gradually pacing up how much you do at a time in order to get out of the boom-and-bust over- or underactivity cycle – the dreaded roller coaster.

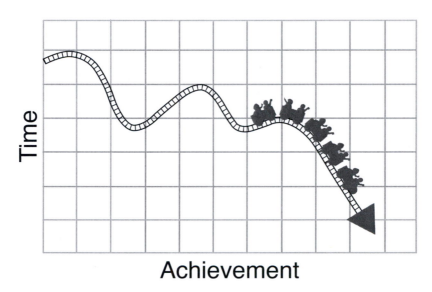

FIGURE 2 Roller coaster

There will be exercise sessions to improve your fitness and stamina, all under the supervision of an expert physiotherapist so you can be confident that nothing will cause you any harm.

You may feel a bit stiff after some of these sessions, as you will gradually be involving muscles that have been resting for a while and may have shortened. However, this is termed *good* pain, related to activity, rather than *bad* pain, related to injury.

> Hurt does not mean harm.

The sessions will be as interactive as possible so you will all be able to produce examples from your own lives and you will find that the more you contribute, the more the programme will help you.

The programme is to help you make changes in your biological, emotional and social responses in order to decrease the negative impact of pain on your life.

Speechmark ⑤ Ⓟ This page may be photocopied for instructional use only © 2014 Keren Fisher and Susan Childs

PROGRAMME RULES

There are a few rules you will need to keep in mind to make sure everyone feels safe and respected.

1. **Confidentiality**. You and your fellow participants may want to disclose aspects of your lives and your private emotions. These need to be kept within the group rooms and not discussed with others outside. You would not like to overhear strangers talking about your personal difficulties.

2. **Punctuality**. Do your best to arrive at every session on time so that the group leader doesn't have to keep going over what has already been covered. You would find this boring. If you are unwell or delayed, try to let the group leader know.

3. **Respectfulness**. Allow everyone a chance to talk in the sessions. Listen when others are making a contribution. You may learn something useful. Be supportive rather than disapproving – you wouldn't like the others to criticise you.

4. **Participation**. It is important to participate in all the group sessions, even if you think they're not for you. Keeping an open mind might allow you to think of new ways of dealing with problems that may have defeated you in the past. Complete the exercises you are given in sessions and as homework. The next task may depend on your responses.

5. **Attentiveness**. Try to keep 'in the moment' about your problems rather than allowing your mind to wander off, regretting actions you have taken in the past or predicting nothing will work in the future.

6. **Curiosity**. Be your own scientist. Try out new things and be enthusiastic to find out the result.

7. **Perseverance**. Some sessions may be hard and upsetting, but keep going and support one another or ask for help from the group leaders.

8. **Medication**. Do not change your normal medication regimen during the programme unless you discuss this with your doctors first. You may find you would like to try reducing some of your drugs but this has to be done gradually and under the supervision of your doctors.

Speechmark ⊚ ℗ This page may be photocopied for instructional use only © 2014 Keren Fisher and Susan Childs

Pain management programme: assessment form

Name................................. Date......... Date of birth.........

Please mark any areas of pain (xxx), pins and needles (///), or numbness (===) on this body map.

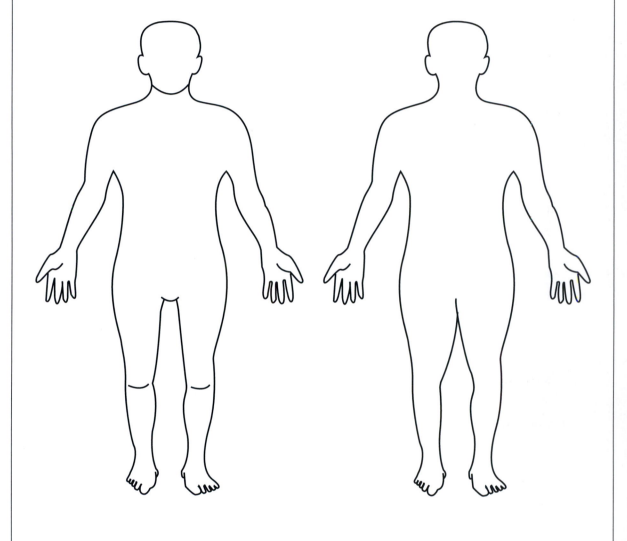

Speechmark ⓟ This page may be photocopied for instructional use only © 2014 Keren Fisher and Susan Childs

Please circle a number along these scales to indicate how much of the items you experience (0 = none, 10 = the worst you can imagine).

How bad is your pain now?

0	1	2	3	4	5	6	7	8	9	10

No pain   Worst pain
                                                                        imaginable

How much pain have you had on average during the last week?

0	1	2	3	4	5	6	7	8	9	10

No pain   Worst pain
                                                                        imaginable

How much distress is your pain causing you now?

0	1	2	3	4	5	6	7	8	9	10

No distress   Worst distress
                                                                        imaginable

How much distress has your pain caused you on average during the last week?

0	1	2	3	4	5	6	7	8	9	10

No distress   Worst distress
                                                                        imaginable

Please answer the following questions:

How long have you had the pain?
How did it start?

Are you awaiting surgery, surgical opinion, injection therapy or other investigations or treatments (e.g. acupuncture, reflexology, osteopathy) in the next six months? If so, what?

Speechmark ⑤ ℗ This page may be photocopied for instructional use only © 2014 Keren Fisher and Susan Childs

Have you had any investigations for your chronic pain? (For example, magnetic resonance imaging, X-ray, nerve conduction studies.) If so, what?

Have you had any operations to treat this pain? If so, what?

What activities help to reduce the pain?

What activities make your pain worse?

Are you currently involved in legal action?

Speechmark ⑤   Ⓟ This page may be photocopied for instructional use only © 2014 Keren Fisher and Susan Childs

OTHER ASSESSMENTS

You may be asked to walk as far as you can in five minutes at your preferred walking pace and taking rests whenever you need to. Experience has shown that walking underpins many other important goals in people's lives, and the distance you can manage in five minutes may increase significantly by the end of the programme. This helps to demonstrate to you how much you have improved by using the strategies you have learned.

You may also be asked to climb some stairs and see how many you can manage in one minute. Your ability to do this also improves by the end of the programme and shows an increase in flexibility and stamina.

The physiotherapy team may ask you to carry out some other activities, depending on the way your particular programme is structured. You will not have to do anything that you find too difficult or scary, but you might try to do just a little to see where you would like to improve.

There might be some questionnaires to fill in from various areas of measurement.

Area of measurement	Suggested questionnaires
Pain quality and intensity	Short Form McGill Pain Questionnaire Numerical rating scales Visual analogue scale
Physical impact of pain	Brief Pain Inventory Roland–Morris Disability Questionnaire Oswestry Disability Index Pain Disability Index
Emotional impact of pain	Beck Depression Inventory Pain Anxiety Symptoms Scale Hospital Anxiety and Depression Scale
Beliefs about pain	Pain Catastrophising Scale Pain Self-Efficacy Scale
Quality of life	SF-36 (36-Item Short Form Health Survey)
Goals	Patient-Specific Functional Scale Canadian Occupational Performance Measure Goal Attainment Scaling (this requires special training)

There are forms for all these questionnaires that can be downloaded for your use from the internet, but for reasons of copyright they cannot be provided here.

TASK

 A TASK FOR YOU

Fill in this table with information you would like to share with the group. Bring this sheet with you on the first day of the programme.

My name or nickname	Where I live	My pain problem in a nutshell	Activities I enjoy	What I hope to gain from the programme

Speechmark This page may be photocopied for instructional use only © 2014 Keren Fisher and Susan Childs

Pain Diaries

Use the pain diary template provided in this section to rate your pain at the beginning of the programme and when there are any significant changes.

1. In the medication column, write down the name and number of any painkiller tablets you take.
2. If you are using a transcutaneous electrical nerve stimulation (TENS) machine, tick the column as appropriate.
3. Record what you are doing every hour during the day.
4. Record how you are feeling each time you fill the diary in.
5. Record your tension and pain levels every hour during the day, and if you wake at night.

PAIN ON A 0–5 RATING SCALE

0 =	No pain
1 =	Very mild
2 =	Mild
3 =	Moderate
4 =	Severe
5 =	Very severe

STRESS OR TENSION ON A 0–5 RATING SCALE

0 =	Calm or relaxed
1 =	Very slightly stressed or tense
2 =	Mildly stressed or tense
3 =	Moderately stressed or tense
4 =	Very stressed or tense
5 =	As stressed as you have ever been

Here is an example of how the pain diary can be filled in.

Time	Medication	TENS	Activity	How are you feeling?	Stress (0–5)	Pain (0–5)
1100	Paracetamol 2 tablets	✓	Washing-up	Frustrated	3	4

DATE _____

Time	Medication	TENS	Activity	How are you feeling?	Stress (0–5)	Pain (0–5)
0600						
0700						
0800						
0900						
1000						
1100						
1200						
1300						
1400						
1500						
1600						
1700						
1800						
1900						
2000						
2100						
2200						
2300						
2400						
0100						
0200						
0300						
0400						
0500						

Speechmark ⓟ This page may be photocopied for instructional use only © 2014 Keren Fisher and Susan Childs

OBSERVING YOUR PAIN: HERE'S A DIARY FOR YOU. RECORDING ASPECTS OF THE PAIN HELPS TO IDENTIFY TRIGGERS AND COPING STRATEGIES.

What was happening before the pain came on or increased?	What was happening at the point when the pain came on or increased?	What happened after the pain came on or increased?

Understanding Chronic Pain: 'All in the Mind' and Other Myths – Models, Anatomy and Theories

Pain is more complex than you might think. It is a complicated system of stages in your whole body. The brain (psyche) and the body (soma) are always working together to try to keep everything in balance. If injury occurs anywhere in the body, the first response of the nervous system is to get excited and send rapid messages (sharp, shooting, acute) sensations up through a series of your nerves in the spinal cord.

They reach the thalamus in the brain. The thalamus then sends an alarm to other brain areas and emergency action might follow. For example, you might remove your thumb quickly if you have bashed it with a hammer.

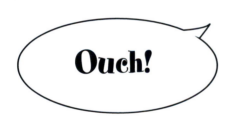

In the meantime, other nerve fibres in the spinal cord send slower sensation messages (dull, aching) up to the brain.

Speechmark Ⓟ This page may be photocopied for instructional use only © 2014 Keren Fisher and Susan Childs

The brain then makes a complicated series of decisions to organise the next stage of response. It causes the injured area to become red and swollen. Blood rushes to the scene full of the ingredients needed to speed up healing. You might feel tired because rest is needed to help the repair process.

TRANSMISSION OF DAMAGE SIGNALS

Figure 1 shows that the problem starts at the area of damage and moves up to the brain.

- *First stage*: damage occurs in a local area of the body. Nerve fibres in the skin respond quickly.
- *Second stage*: special nerve fibres transmit injury or danger signals through the spinal cord by a system of 'gates' or synapses.
- *Third stage*: (a) rapid and (b) slower signals arrive at the thalamus in the brain and are transmitted to other brain areas.
- *Fourth stage*: the brain makes decisions about the danger messages and sends information back down the spinal cord.

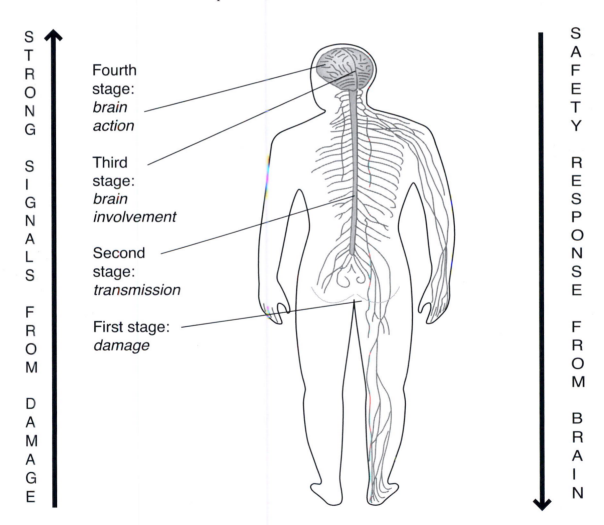

FIGURE 1 Transmission of damage signals

Speechmark Ⓟ This page may be photocopied for instructional use only © 2014 Keren Fisher and Susan Childs

SYNAPSE

Nerve fibres in the spine send chemicals (called neurotransmitters) to carry the injury signals to one another via synapses or 'gates'.

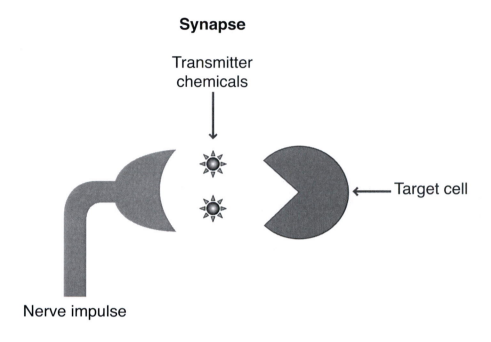

FIGURE 2 Synapse

The signals are noxious (nasty) and travel up the spinal cord to the brain.

Within the brain the pathway is still complex and occurs in stages. The signals are registered in the thalamus by a process called *nociception*. The thalamus is a major relay station in the centre of the brain.

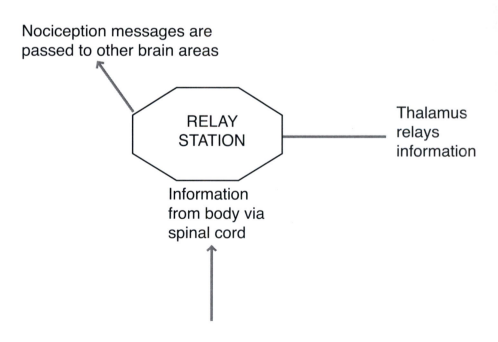

FIGURE 3 Nociception

 Speechmark ⑤ Ⓟ This page may be photocopied for instructional use only © 2014 Keren Fisher and Susan Childs

MEMORY AND EMOTIONAL MESSAGES

The memory and emotional parts of the brain – the *limbic system* – get involved to compare these signals with pain memories and emotions that you may have experienced previously.

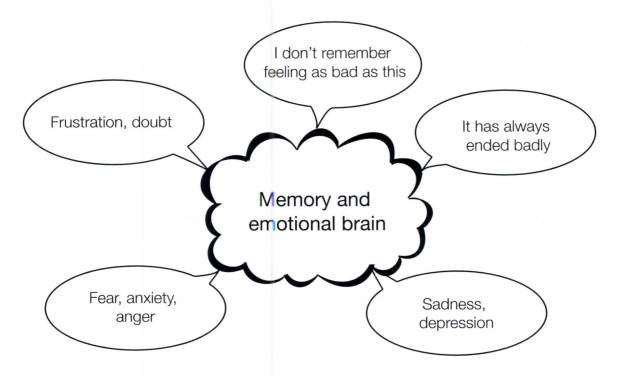

Messages are now passed to the thinking brain – the cortex. This will add thoughts like, *'I'm not able to do the things I used to enjoy'.*

Speechmark Ⓟ This page may be photocopied for instructional use only © 2014 Keren Fisher and Susan Childs 19

TASK

    A TASK FOR YOU

The decision about the danger value of *nociception* messages depends on a lot of information already stored in your brain as a result of past experience.

Emotional responses and *memories* are added in the limbic system to the noxious signals and then passed on to the cortex where *thoughts* and *beliefs* are also added to give the total pain experience. This complex interaction within the stages of the brain produces pain.

What are your typical emotions and memories when you experience pain?

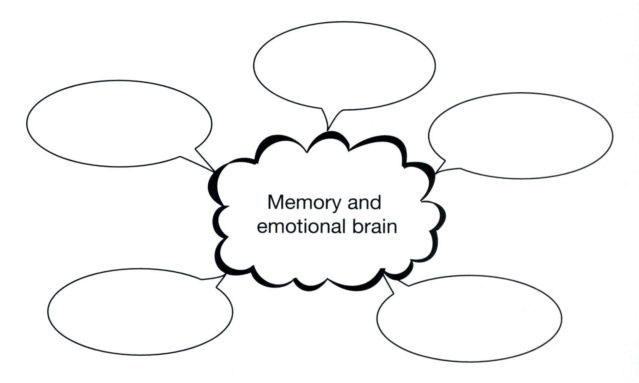

Fill in some thoughts from your thinking brain about this situation:

_____

_____

_____

_____

Speechmark ⑤ ℗ This page may be photocopied for instructional use only © 2014 Keren Fisher and Susan Childs

NOCICEPTION VERSUS PAIN

The thinking brain area of the *cortex*, particularly the frontal region, decides how dangerous the noxious signals coming from the thalamus really are.

At the end of all these processes, when the noxious signals have passed up through the spine and brain stem, the major relay station (the thalamus), the emotional and memory system (the limbic system) and the thinking brain (the cortex), the experience becomes labelled as *pain*.

This is what is meant when people say that **pain occurs in the brain**.

> *Nociception* becomes ***pain*** only after the thinking brain has put all the information together.

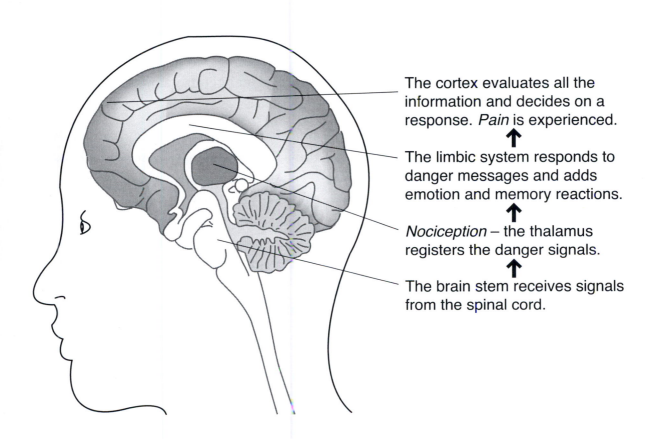

The cortex evaluates all the information and decides on a response. *Pain* is experienced.

⬆

The limbic system responds to danger messages and adds emotion and memory reactions.

⬆

Nociception – the thalamus registers the danger signals.

⬆

The brain stem receives signals from the spinal cord.

Speechmark ⓢ Ⓟ This page may be photocopied for instructional use only © 2014 Keren Fisher and Susan Childs

PAINFUL SYMPTOMS: A TWO-WAY HIGHWAY TO AND FROM THE BRAIN

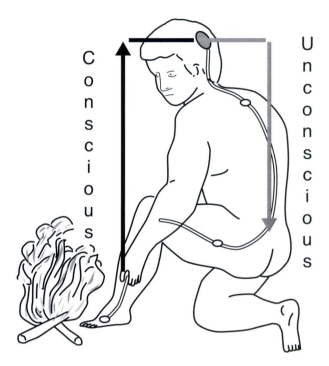

This famous picture shows that pain is a *conscious* experience.

It is *conscious* because you can:
- see the injury
- feel the pain
- possibly hear or smell it.

However, pain is also an *unconscious* experience.

It is *unconscious* because the brain sends down strong messages to make you take care and prevent further injury. This is helpful in the early stages but it is not helpful later on. Because these responses are unconscious, you might not be aware of how much they influence your reactions.

The response you actually make to the pain will depend on the context in which you experience it.

> If you are lying in the middle of the road, having been knocked off your bicycle, you will move to a safe place first – perhaps even before you feel any pain. Your thinking brain has decided to make your safety a priority over responding to your injuries.

The cortex is responsible for evaluating all the input information and making the output decision. So, the pain that is felt is the result of the balance between the up-coming information and the down-going messages. These try to prevent overactivity in the spinal cord or further injury. This is all happening outside of your consciousness, *so you are unaware of all these processes.*

 Speechmark ⑤ ℗ This page may be photocopied for instructional use only © 2014 Keren Fisher and Susan Childs

GETTING BACK INTO BALANCE

Other areas of the nervous system – mainly in the base of the brain, the *brain stem* – will help the situation get back to normal by sending *safety response* messages down to the spinal cord.

Some of these chemical messengers have names that might be familiar to you. They are *serotonin* and *endorphins* – feel-good chemicals that help sleep and good mood.

They are responsible for telling the thalamus that the situation is under control.

> Usually, the original injury heals and the damaged area goes back to normal. The gates in the spine close and the excited nerve fibres stop sending danger signals. The situation returns to a balanced state, which is nature's comfort zone.

This is the normal pattern of events that follows from an *acute* injury.

ACUTE VERSUS CHRONIC PAIN

Unfortunately, for reasons we do not yet understand, sometimes pain will continue to be felt months after the injury has healed. Time has passed and the situation is now persistent or *chronic*.

> 'Chronic' means it's been going a long time, rather than referring to how bad it feels.

Acute pain
1. Sudden onset
2. Closely associated with injury
3. Accompanied by visible signs of injury (e.g. swelling, redness)
4. Experienced in a specific body part
5. Progressively improves with healing

Chronic pain
1. Prolonged onset over weeks or months
2. No longer accompanied by signs of injury
3. Widespread over body regions
4. Varies with emotional or social context
5. No predictable time course

All the transmission processes are still active, damage messages are still firing along the spinal nerves and alerting the brain to danger even though the injury has cleared up.

CHANGES THAT OCCUR IN CHRONIC PAIN

The longer the nerve fibres go on firing, the wider the spinal gates open up to allow more and more noxious information through.

- Instead of just the pathways that carried the original information, there are now whole highways sending messages to the brain.
- The pathways start to *steal the routes* that used to be used for other information. Touch sensations start to feel like pain and other feelings in different parts of the body also get added to the pain mixture. The downward routes for the feel-good chemicals get taken over too.
- The thalamus is now in constant **danger** mode and the decision-making part of the brain (the cortex) spends a lot of its time trying to evaluate what to do.

This means it is harder for you to attend to other tasks.

- Emotional reactions become more extreme and thought processes become preoccupied with beliefs about the hopelessness of the situation.
- This sets up a vicious circle of helplessness thoughts, leading to despairing emotions, leading to reduced ability to send useful action messages down the spine. This will lead to increased danger messages coming up and an increased belief that the injury is ongoing.

A particularly appropriate label is given to this situation:

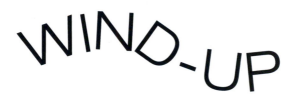

Sensitisation of the nervous system

Pain is experienced in the brain but the whole nervous system has become sensitised and overexcited. This is not because you have a particular personality type, or a mental illness or a habit of exaggerating your problems, but it is the result of long-term firing of networks of nerve fibres that have learned to wire themselves together.

Speechmark ⓅThis page may be photocopied for instructional use only © 2014 Keren Fisher and Susan Childs

EVER-INCREASING PATHWAYS GET ADDED TO THE PAIN NETWORK

The pain network gradually spreads over a wider area of the brain. As the pain persists more emotions and beliefs get added to the total sensation.

If you had an injury in the past that led to serious consequences, then this has set up a *belief* pathway (*that activity made my pain worse; I must avoid it in future*) and possibly also a *fear* pathway (*I'm afraid to do that again in case I get worse*). These pathways will tend to get activated if you experience any new pain.

> These pathways will *share information* with the pain pathway. They have the power to make the pain seem different at different times, depending on the strength of the fear or beliefs. The brain will then respond to the messages from the thalamus and to many other cues as well.

The pain situation now looks a bit like the diagram in Figure 4.

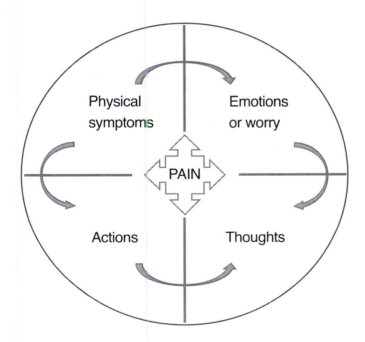

FIGURE 4 The pain situation

Some of the triggers for the pain pathway to become more active might be:

- social context (more pain might be experienced in the presence of some people than in the presence of others – even seeing someone else in pain might activate the pain network)
- previous experience of dealing with discomfort
- expectation that it will all end in a catastrophe (e.g. It's never going to get better. I'll become totally disabled.)
- anxiety, depression, stress.

A TASK FOR YOU

Write details of the components of your pain problem in this diagram.

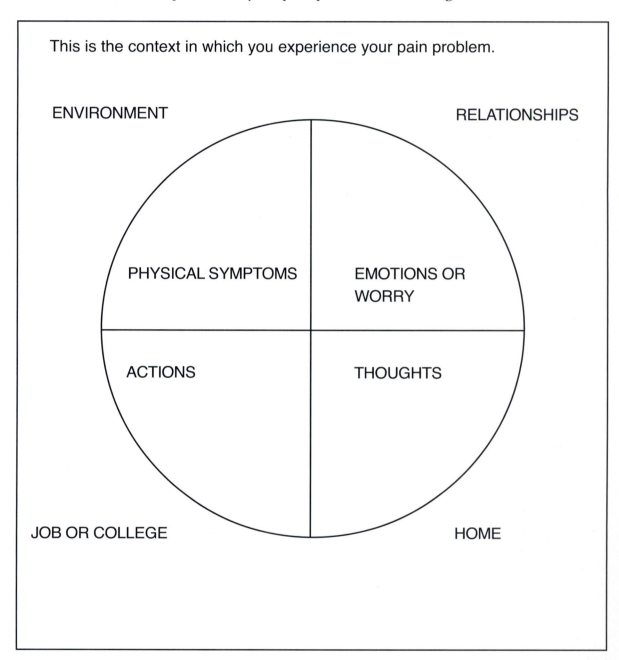

This is the context in which you experience your pain problem.

ENVIRONMENT

RELATIONSHIPS

PHYSICAL SYMPTOMS

EMOTIONS OR WORRY

ACTIONS

THOUGHTS

JOB OR COLLEGE

HOME

What have you noticed about this problem when you look at it in this way?

_____

_____

_____

_____

Speechmark P This page may be photocopied for instructional use only © 2014 Keren Fisher and Susan Childs

INFORMATION LEADS TO LEARNING OF NEW NETWORKS

With all the extra information, the brain loses its ability to keep focused on the specific noxious sensations and this leads to more routes and faster transmission between the stages.

The growing spread of brain cells recruited to the pain experience leads to changes in the nerve fibres themselves.

> They have *learned* to become more sensitive and less specific in their readiness to respond to sensations in the skin. This is something your nervous system is doing – you are still unaware of it all.

It is obvious that the brain can learn. You presumably know more now than you did as a baby. New wiring takes place to create rapid pathways to give you access to information you use all the time.

If you move house, you can easily learn the new route to the train station because new networks get wired together quickly. The brain has usefully rewired the home-to-station network.

> This situation is the same for pain. New pain networks develop as a result of frequent firing of the nociception messengers all getting wired together with the thoughts, emotions and memory reactions. The brain actually changes.

This isn't so surprising, but what we are only just realising is that the spinal cord nerves can learn too. Nerve fibres that usually carry different messages from the skin get wired together and the sensations they normally transmit become involved in sending damage signals up to the brain.

> Usually the fibres have 'gates' between them that close once an injury has healed. The fibres return to working fairly separately. After chronic pain changes have occurred, the gates stay open and then the different fibres get caught up in nociception networks.

Figure 5 represents what we think is happening in the spinal nerves.

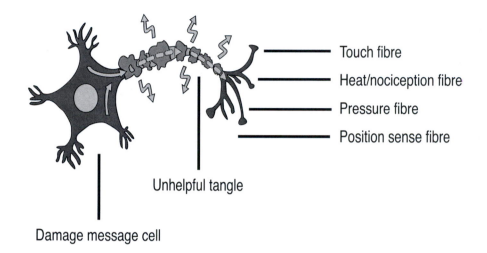

FIGURE 5 Spinal nerve

DOWNWARD ROUTES GET TAKEN OVER

If you could 'hear' the communication between the chemical messengers in the spine, it might sound a bit like this conversation.

Noxious Alarm Transmitting Signals (*NATS*): Must run, there's more information coming in that I have to pass up to Thalamus.

Easy-Going Safety Signals (*EGSS*): No hurry, there's no real danger.

NATS: That's not true. There's new information from different body parts all the time. I must tell Thalamus. It's probably important.

EGSS: You keep crowding me out. I'm trying to tell you, there's no real danger.

NATS: More information is coming. I need more pathways to deal with it. Please move out of the way.

EGSS: I wish you'd pay attention when I tell you there *is no new danger*. Now you've taken over quite a lot of my space.

NATS: Sorry, can't hear you. Have to run.

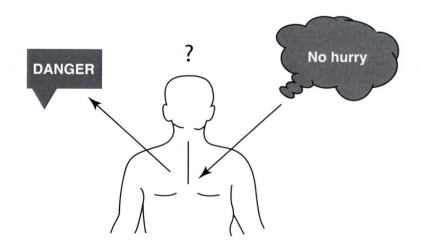

Speechmark (P) This page may be photocopied for instructional use only © 2014 Keren Fisher and Susan Childs

This wind-up in the spinal cord has changed the behaviour of the cells themselves.

> This situation can explain why treatments such as operations to remove the previously damaged body part do not always reduce the pain. Even after a limb has been amputated the original pain might still be firing off in the sensitised nervous system. *The surgery itself has not been able to correct the rewiring that has taken place.* The rewiring is not useful but it has happened automatically.

THE MANAGEMENT OF ACUTE AND CHRONIC PAIN IS DIFFERENT

In the *acute* situation, the priority is to promote healing as quickly as possible and prevent the pain becoming chronic. The emergency signals, the open spinal gates and the excitation in the nervous system are all there to alert the brain to take rapid action and prevent further injury.

Once the pain has become *chronic*, these responses are no longer useful and a whole range of new techniques need to take their place in order to try to reverse the changes in the nervous system.

Management of acute pain
APRICOTS can help you remember

Management of chronic pain
GRAPES can help you remember

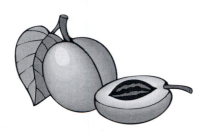

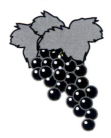

Avoid the activity that caused the injury
Protect the part to prevent more damage
Raise the injured part
Ice the area to reduce swelling
Compress the injured part with a bandage
Opiates (painkillers) – take for a *short* while
Take time out from normal commitments
Seek more medical advice if necessary

Goals to achieve more things you value
Relaxation techniques to reduce wind-up
Activity to enhance your life
Pacing to stop over- or underactivity cycles
Exercise to increase fitness and confidence
Self-help rather than unhelpful treatments

Speechmark P This page may be photocopied for instructional use only © 2014 Keren Fisher and Susan Childs

WHAT WILL HELP?

There are a few ways to try to modify the oversensitivity of the nerve cells. Medication and other physical treatments are some, but the most successful at present seems to be to train the brain to reduce the added emotion and thought messages. This will help the brain to discriminate new from familiar nociception.

Pain management programmes are quite good at starting this process. They can help you understand the changes in the nerve networks that occurred outside of your awareness. This will help to wind down the sensitivity in the nervous system and will start to set up a *confidence* pathway in place of a *fear* pathway. This, in turn, will help the body regain more normal movement and this will reduce anxiety and catastrophic beliefs.

> Pain management programmes help you to regain more of the life you want.

You can learn to use deliberate techniques to bring the system back into balance. This can help you move from the struggle for control to a better quality of life with more of the activities you value even if there's still some pain.

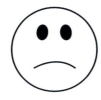

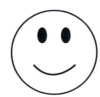

PAIN MANAGEMENT STRATEGIES

Pre pain management programme
- Suffering with persistent pain
- Life dominated by pain
- Activities associated with catastrophic thoughts
- Avoidance of movement
- Life goals abandoned
- Ineffective strategies to control pain
- Mood and activity in a boom-and-bust roller-coaster cycle
- Where you are is *not* where you wanted to be

Post pain management programme
- Living the life you want
- Awareness of thoughts, actions and emotions
- Valued activities become possible again
- You become willing to embrace the bad with the good
- Effective management strategies stop the roller coaster
- Understanding your personal rate of improvement helps you plan to get where you want to be

Speechmark ⓢ ℗ This page may be photocopied for instructional use only © 2014 Keren Fisher and Susan Childs

A TASK FOR YOU

What are the differences between acute and chronic pain? Put a tick in the right columns.

Characteristic of pain	Acute	Chronic
Progressively improves		
Prolonged		
Specific		
Sudden onset		
Unpredictable		
Varies with social or emotional context		
Visible injury		
Widespread		

Treatment strategy	Acute	Chronic
Activity		
Avoiding further injury		
Compression		
Exercise		
Goals		
Ice		
Opiates – short term		
Pacing		
Protection		
Raising injured part		
Relaxation		
Seeking more advice		
Self-help		
Taking time out		

Speechmark Ⓟ This page may be photocopied for instructional use only © 2014 Keren Fisher and Susan Childs

Understanding Diagnosis and Interventions

Trying to diagnose the *cause* of chronic pain is like trying to extinguish the candle that started the fire while the house is burning down.

So many changes have occurred in the time you have been suffering from persistent pain that it is now very difficult to identify the original incident. This may be no longer relevant or even recognisable. Medical treatments for chronic pain have limited success and at present there is no known 'cure' or recognised way of reversing the nervous system changes that occur as pain messages become established in the spinal cord and brain.

Imagine yourself as the diagram in Figure 1a. All the doctor knows about you to start with are your symptoms – those are the points you complain of: the pain, fatigue, muscle weakness and the other things you feel. These are private *subjective experiences* – no one else can know about them unless you tell them. In order to understand more about the cause or pathology, the doctor needs to find out about the *objective signs* of the problem that explain your symptoms and may then order investigations. This is appropriate in the acute phase, but if a diagnosis cannot be reached, the situation eventually changes to chronic (*see* Figure 1b) and treatment has to focus on the symptoms.

Speechmark ⑤ Ⓟ This page may be photocopied for instructional use only © 2014 Keren Fisher and Susan Childs

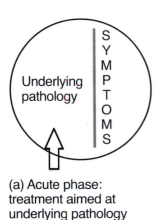

(a) Acute phase:
treatment aimed at
underlying pathology

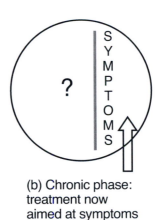

(b) Chronic phase:
treatment now
aimed at symptoms

FIGURE 1 Pain: **(a)** acute phase and **(b)** chronic phase

The problem with most investigations such as X-ray, computerised tomography or magnetic resonance imaging scans is that they can tell us what things look like – normal or abnormal – but not what they do or how they behave. Even when there are abnormalities on the scans, these may not explain the reason for or even relate to your pain at all. Many people have abnormal X-rays but do not experience pain.

Confusing results from medical examinations may lead to assumptions about the problem being 'psychosomatic' or, worse, 'all in the mind'. This sets you and your doctor on a collision course, which is less than helpful.

TASK

    A TASK FOR YOU

Consider whether a diagnosis is important or not – fill in the grid.

Have you had a diagnosis?	
If yes, in what way was it helpful?	How did that affect how you manage the problem?
If no, how did you feel?	How did that affect how you manage the problem?

Speechmark   This page may be photocopied for instructional use only © 2014 Keren Fisher and Susan Childs

MEDICAL TREATMENTS AND OTHER INTERVENTIONS

Drugs are undoubtedly helpful, but they have side effects and unfortunately they are not often 'smart'. Rather than targeting only the nerves that are continually transmitting signals about **danger** they slow everything down, including your brain. This may result in you feeling drowsy or dizzy and make it difficult for you to get on with your valued activities. Then the whole problem seems like it's going in the wrong direction.

There are four main classes of drugs that are used for pain (other than over-the-counter pain-killers such as paracetamol or aspirin). These are:

1. *opiates* (e.g. morphine and tramadol)
2. *non-steroidal anti-inflammatory drugs* (e.g. ibuprofen, diclofenac)
3. *antidepressants*, in lower doses than are used for depression (e.g. amitriptyline, duloxetine)
4. *anticonvulsants* (e.g. gabapentin, pregabalin) (nerve pain seems like 'local epilepsy').

They all need to be taken exactly as advised by your doctor. Higher doses won't work better and may be harmful. Excessive doses of even paracetamol and aspirin are toxic to your liver and stomach and can be fatal.

Surgical operations can be helpful if the results of the investigations – the signs – match your symptoms, so there is a good chance of putting the problem right without creating a new one. However, if that were the simple answer, you would not have chronic pain now.

Other kinds of treatment may not be available on the NHS. This is because there may be little evidence of their effectiveness. The National Institute for Health and Care Excellence distributes guidelines to help the NHS to know what has been proved to be useful and cost-effective.

There may be other procedures that some practitioners use and which have questionable relevance and can only be provided privately for that reason. You have to pay, but there may be no evidence of any benefit. £ £ £ £ $ $ $ $ € € € €   ¥ ¥ ¥ ¥

Even treatments such as massage may help you to feel better temporarily but do little to change the problem in the long term.

In the end, it may be best not to depend on others but to look at how you are managing your pain and lifestyle for yourself. Here you have two options – choose the one you prefer.

Offer conflicting advice	You take control
Take control away	Own goals are achieved
Have differing opinions	Unhelpful strategies are discontinued
Expect quick results	Relaxation is practised
Resort to strong medicines	Self-directed pacing is helpful
Stress you further	Exercise is increased
	Life gets better
	Feelings improve

Speechmark ⓈⒻ ⓟ This page may be photocopied for instructional use only © 2014 Keren Fisher and Susan Childs

TASK

    A TASK FOR YOU

List the treatments you have already had and consider their effects.

Type of treatment	Short-term benefit?	Long-term benefit?	Any harmful effects?	NHS or private?

What did you learn from this exercise?

_____

_____

_____

_____

Speechmark P This page may be photocopied for instructional use only © 2014 Keren Fisher and Susan Childs

THE PROBLEM OF 'ILLNESS'

Would you classify a long-term pain problem as an illness? If you know other people with chronic pain, ask them which of these two boxes they see themselves fitting into.

ILL

WELL

This probably did not work very well, as pain doesn't fit this type of dichotomy – it's more like a continuum. Where do you see yourself on an ill–well continuum?

Speechmark P This page may be photocopied for instructional use only © 2014 Keren Fisher and Susan Childs

TASK

     A TASK FOR YOU

Ask other people where they think they fit along the line of an ill–well continuum. Compare their estimate with your own.

ILL -- WELL

Most people with chronic pain see themselves as quite well most of the time but they might get worse when they have flare-ups.

The point of pain management programmes is to help people move as far as they can to the well end of the continuum and to use self-management strategies to get over flare-ups as quickly as possible. You can join together with other people with similar problems and support one another to build self-confidence. This gives you the skills needed to take on previously abandoned, or new, valued activities. You gain a sense of your own health and learn to schedule your activities so that you become your own case manager.

How you live with a chronic health problem can change its effects and sometimes even the course of the problem itself.

Speechmark P This page may be photocopied for instructional use only © 2014 Keren Fisher and Susan Childs

MOVING FROM ILL TO WELL

Let's look at some other long-term health problems. What are some of the things people can do during a flare-up to move themselves back to the well end of the ill–well continuum?

Diabetes
Identify triggers
      Check appropriate use of medicines
          Use relaxation techniques
             Continue with exercise for fitness
                Continue to achieve small goals

ILL --- WELL
Flare-up   ⟶

Asthma
Identify triggers
      Check appropriate use of medicines
          Use relaxation techniques
             Continue with exercise for fitness
                Continue to achieve small goals

ILL --- WELL
Flare-up   ⟶

Arthritis
Identify triggers
      Check appropriate use of medicines
          Use relaxation techniques
             Continue with exercise for fitness
                Continue to achieve small goals

ILL --- WELL
Flare-up   ⟶

Chronic pain – the pattern is the same
Identify triggers
      Check appropriate use of medicines
          Use relaxation techniques
             Continue with exercise for fitness
                Continue to achieve small goals

ILL --- WELL
Flare-up   ⟶

Speechmark ⓟ This page may be photocopied for instructional use only © 2014 Keren Fisher and Susan Childs

Beginning the Process of Change in Negative Thinking in Chronic Pain Management: A Cognitive Behavioural Therapy Approach

This section is about understanding the influence of thoughts on reactions. It is about identifying the thoughts that accompany some of the emotions you feel about your pain situation and how they influence your responses.

People dealing with chronic pain sometimes describe feelings of depression, anxiety, anger, frustration, irritability and other such negative moods. They also often complain about achieving fewer of the things that are important to them. Why is this?

Why do some chronic pain sufferers experience more low moods and reduced activity than others?

The answer to this question is more complex than you might suppose.

Consider this example.

> You are sitting alone at home at night. Suddenly you hear a loud explosion in the street outside. You immediately feel extremely *afraid*. You might move quickly to a safer room before you dare to look out of the window. You might ring your friend and report that what you think you heard was someone shooting a gun in your street. *'It's possible'*, you say, *'Gun crime is on the increase.'*

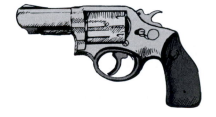

> Alternatively, you might pay no attention to the loud explosion and feel *calm*. You continue reading your book. Later, when your son comes home, you might

Speechmark ⑤ Ⓟ This page may be photocopied for instructional use only © 2014 Keren Fisher and Susan Childs

say, 'I heard you go down the street. You really must get your exhaust fixed and stop it backfiring.'

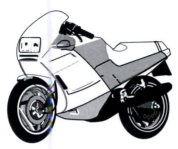

INTERPRETATION OF EVENTS IS THE KEY TO REACTION

The difference between your reactions depends on the interpretation of an event such as a loud noise. The emotion of fear and the behaviour of moving out of the way would follow completely logically from the thought, 'The noise was caused by a gunshot.' Similarly, the thought, 'That's my son's bike backfiring again', would lead logically to calm reactions, since you are used to hearing it.

The situation is the same but the thought about it has led to different responses. Your central control brain (cortex) has organised the information and produced a consistent set of responses.

Thought	→	Emotion	→	Behaviour
Gunshot	→	Fear, panic	→	Hide and phone for help
Bike backfiring	→	Calmness	→	Continue reading

Similarly, with the situation of chronic pain, thoughts can influence emotions and behavioural responses.

There are four parts to a situation:
A. the event itself
B. your thoughts
C. your emotions
D. your behavioural response.

Usually people are only aware of parts A, C and D, but it is part B, your thoughts about the situation, that determines how you feel and react. You need to take a step back and analyse the interpretation you have attached to the event. Then you can begin to tell your central control brain to change your response.

> Negative interpretations will produce unpleasant emotions and reduce your chances of behaviour change. Neutral or more positive interpretations can improve behaviour change.

Speechmark Ⓟ This page may be photocopied for instructional use only © 2014 Keren Fisher and Susan Childs

THOUGHTS ABOUT THE PAIN SITUATION INFLUENCE EMOTION AND BEHAVIOUR

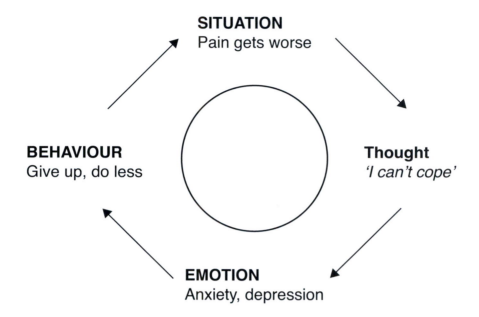

FIGURE 1 Thought: *'I can't cope'*

Alternatively, a coping thought might lead to an improved outcome.

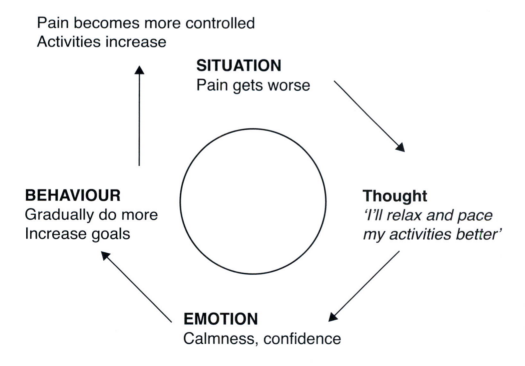

FIGURE 2 Coping thought: *'I'll relax and pace my activities better'*

Speechmark P This page may be photocopied for instructional use only © 2014 Keren Fisher and Susan Childs

THE DIFFERENCE BETWEEN EMOTIONS AND THOUGHTS

Cognitive behavioural therapy (CBT) teaches that there is a crucial difference between thoughts and emotions. An emotional reaction to a triggering event is determined by the thoughts that are associated with it. CBT spends a lot of time getting people to recognise this process, so that the *thoughts* can be examined for their influence on the *feelings*.

Feelings are emotions or moods. Fear, anger, sadness, happiness, guilt, shame, pity, envy are *emotions*.

Feelings can be described in one word and some-times it is useful to measure their intensity on a scale from 0 to 100 per cent, where 0 per cent is none of the feeling and 100 per cent is a very strong amount.

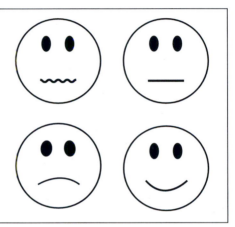

Thoughts are beliefs, images and memories. Thoughts may take the form of words or pictures and will answer the question: *'What was in my mind when I noticed my emotions change?'* They may need several words to describe them. You can't measure thoughts in the same way as emotions, but you can rate how much you think they are true.

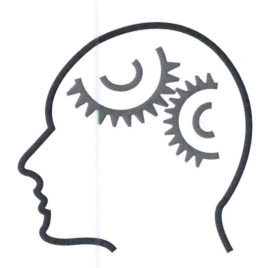

TASK

     A TASK FOR YOU

Tick the appropriate column for each item according to whether you think it is an emotion or a thought.

> *Beware*: The word 'feel' is often used incorrectly to imply a strong belief. In CBT the word 'feel' needs to be kept for describing emotions. This helps to keep the difference clear in your mind.

		Emotion	Thought
1	I feel anxious		
2	I feel panicky quite often		
3	I feel I won't enjoy things like I used to		
4	I feel something terrible is about to happen		
5	I feel nothing ever goes right now		
6	I feel sad most of the time		
7	I feel I'm useless now		
8	I feel I can't do even simple things like I used to		
9	I feel my friends won't include me in their plans		
10	I feel irritable		
11	I feel depressed		
12	I feel I'm a burden on my family		
13	I feel nervous		
14	I feel angry that the doctor doesn't help me		
15	I feel frustrated that I don't get better		
16	I feel I should be quicker or I'll lose my job		
17	I feel guilty about needing help		
18	I feel I'm no good for anything any more		
19	I feel I'm not able to carry on		
20	I feel worried about the future		

If it is difficult to get the point of this exercise, try crossing out 'feel' and put 'think' instead. This will only work for the statements that are really thoughts – the rest are emotions. This will make the distinction clearer.

Speechmark   P   This page may be photocopied for instructional use only © 2014 Keren Fisher and Susan Childs

THOUGHTS ARE PROBABLY THE EASIEST PART OF A SITUATION TO CHANGE

Imagine the situation of waiting for a bus that has been delayed. You *feel* anxious, frustrated and annoyed. Your *behavioural response* might be to pace about or to complain to your fellow passengers. Your *thoughts* might be: *'Why can't they sort this route out? This is a disaster. I shall be late for work again. I might lose my job.'*

The more your thoughts focus on a bad outcome, the more powerful your emotions will get and the more agitated your behaviour will become. Your central control (cortex) will organise a stronger output consistent with the strength of the information it receives from your interpretation of the event. Consider your options.

Is it easy to change:		Yes	No
… the situation?	Bus delayed		✓
… your emotional reaction that follows from your interpretation of the situation?	Anxiety or frustration or annoyance		✓
… your behaviour that follows from your emotion?	Pacing about or complaining		✓
… your thought or interpretation?	This is a disaster	✓	

You could decide to change your thought or interpretation to: *'I'll text my boss with an explanation and try to make sure I don't miss my deadline.'* Then logically your emotion will become calmer (although possibly still a bit annoyed) and your behaviour will become more relaxed.

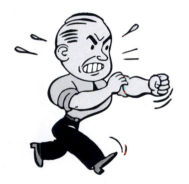 → Change interpretation of situation →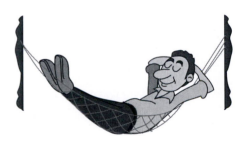

Speechmark Ⓟ This page may be photocopied for instructional use only © 2014 Keren Fisher and Susan Childs

THE PROCESS OF CHANGE

Figure 3 shows how your thoughts will influence the central control system in the cortex to produce your behavioural response. Negative thoughts will produce fewer useful behaviours than neutral thoughts do.

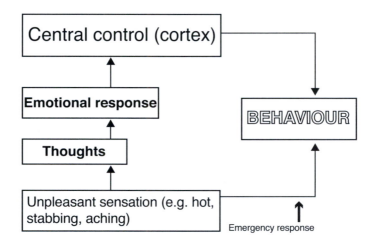

FIGURE 3 The influence of thoughts

Thoughts can influence behaviour: a pain management example

In a pain management programme you might be asked to *start some gentle stretches*. You have done exercises before and are now convinced they will hurt you. *Your emotion will be fear or frustration*. What will be your behavioural response? Probably you will join in only very reluctantly and you will move very cautiously.

Take a step back and ask yourself:

> 'What was in my mind when I started to feel anxious about what the therapist was asking me to do?'

Perhaps your answer to this question is something like:

> 'I know this will be bad for me. It always makes things worse.'

This negative thought will automatically influence your anxious reaction and cautious response.

Your thoughts are the easiest part to change. You might decide to interpret the new instruction for stretches as:

> 'I'll see if it'll be different this time.'

Then your response will be more like that of a *curious scientist* who doesn't know the outcome but is keen to find it out!

 Speechmark ⑤   ⓟ This page may be photocopied for instructional use only © 2014 Keren Fisher and Susan Childs

A TASK FOR YOU

Mood Log 1

Attempt to catch some negative thoughts that occur to you in the next few days and jot them down on this form. You may only be aware of your emotional reaction to the situation to start with, but think about the way you have interpreted it, which is really the cause of the reaction.

Then you will see the order is really:

A. the situation itself
B. your thoughts
C. your feelings
D. your behavioural response.

A

Step 1: Describe the upsetting **situation or event**.

B

Step 3: **Thoughts**. What did you think at the time of this event?
How true would you rate these thoughts? (On a scale from 0 to 100 per cent)

C

Step 2: **Feelings**. What emotion did you feel? (For example, angry, sad, anxious)
How much? (On a scale from 0 to 100 per cent)
Remember to use only one word for each feeling.

D

Step 4: **Behavioural response**. What did you do?
Was it helpful?

 P This page may be photocopied for instructional use only © 2014 Keren Fisher and Susan Childs   47

DISCRIMINATING FACTS AND INTERPRETATIONS

Most automatic thoughts have a grain of truth in them but are so distorted that they are inaccurate. The first step is to try to sort out the facts from your interpretation of an event.

Facts are information you can prove, while interpretations tell you how someone has responded to it.

A fact might be: '*This book has 600 pages.*'

An interpretation would be: '*This book is really boring.*'

Someone else might interpret the book as '*really thrilling.*'

The interpretations 'boring' and 'thrilling' are opinions and will vary according to the circumstances of the people who make the evaluation. They don't affect the truth of the statement that the book has 600 pages.

It is not always easy to spot when a statement is true and unbiased by opinion and when it is not, especially when you feel low or anxious. These moods will tend to make *negative interpretations* come into your mind automatically, and it might not occur to you to question whether they are facts or opinions.

In order to discriminate facts and interpretations, you could consider that *facts* relate to what you can *see, hear or touch* about a situation. Interpretations are thoughts that relate to how good or bad a situation is.

For example, you might think: '*When the weather is cold it is too difficult to do my exercises.*' You might believe this is a fact, but if you ask yourself, '*Can I see, hear or touch something about this thought?*' you will probably conclude that it is actually your opinion.

You could ask yourself, '*Was this thought helpful in achieving my task?*' If not, you could try an alternative interpretation, such as: '*I could wear more clothes and have a hot shower so that I can keep up my exercise regimen.*'

Speechmark ⓢ Ⓟ This page may be photocopied for instructional use only © 2014 Keren Fisher and Susan Childs

A TASK FOR YOU

Decide whether each statement in this scenario is a fact or an interpretation and put a tick in the appropriate column.

> Mary has a diagnosis of chronic back pain. She lives a long way from town and shopping is difficult for her. It takes her a long time. Her daughter comes to stay and Mary finds the situation stressful. She has a pain flare-up and believes it's intolerable. She discusses the situation with her daughter and they agree to share the shopping.

	Statement	Fact	Interpretation
1	Mary has chronic back pain		
2	She lives a long way from town		
3	Shopping is difficult for her		
4	It takes her a long time		
5	Her daughter comes to stay		
6	Mary finds the situation stressful		
7	She has a pain flare-up		
8	'It's intolerable'		
9	She discusses the situation with her daughter		
10	They agree to share the shopping		

Mary has medical evidence that she has chronic pain and has flare-ups. Statements 1 and 7 are facts. You could see or hear evidence for statements 2, 4, 5, 9 and 10, so these are facts. The others are Mary's interpretation.

TASK

● ● ●   A TASK FOR YOU

Try this exercise using an example from your own life.

The situation was:

What happened next?

What was your response?

Decide if there is anything you can see, hear or touch about your answers. Then fill in this form with the statements you have made about your situation and your response and tick the appropriate column.

	Statement	Fact	Interpretation
1			
2			
3			
4			
5			
6			
7 etc			

Speechmark   P   This page may be photocopied for instructional use only © 2014 Keren Fisher and Susan Childs

IDENTIFYING NEGATIVE THINKING DISTORTIONS IN CHRONIC PAIN

When you have pain that reduces your ability to achieve the things you want, it is useful to identify ways in which *thoughts* are too focused on a negative outcome. If the thoughts do not fit the *facts* of the situation, they are usually

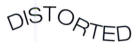

This process of distortion means that negative thoughts take on a life of their own without your being aware that they are doing it. They come automatically without your having to conjure them up. These negative automatic thoughts will lead to unhelpful emotions and responses.

You might only be aware of negative feelings (emotions) such as anxiety, sadness, anger or depression, but these alert you to considering the thoughts that may have set them off. Take a step back from your feelings and ask yourself:

'What was in my mind when I started to feel like this?'

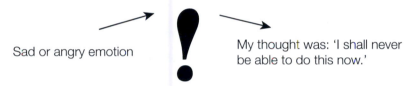

Sad or angry emotion

My thought was: 'I shall never be able to do this now.'

Distorted negative automatic thoughts can be associated with increases in your pain, distress and disability.

There are several ways in which negative automatic thoughts can be distorted and affect your emotions and behaviour, but most of them result in reducing your motivation to carry out your valued activities. When this happens, you tend to lead a life dominated by pain instead of achieving what you really want. Valued activities (things you want to do to improve your life) are overbalanced by the weight of negative thoughts and feelings about the things you have to do to stay alive. *Changing the negative thoughts will allow for a better balance.*

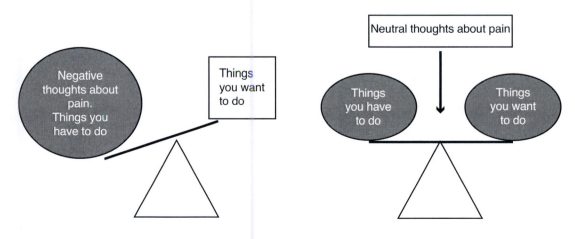

Speechmark Ⓟ This page may be photocopied for instructional use only © 2014 Keren Fisher and Susan Childs

IDENTIFYING DISTORTIONS IN THOUGHTS

Negative thoughts have several characteristics but they may be *interpretations* of events based on opinion rather than *fact*.

The thoughts you have about your pain may appear to be true and occur to you frequently but they probably contain **distortions** that keep your mood low. This will prevent your using your best possible coping responses.

PUDDING can help you identify negative automatic thoughts.

Plausible: it doesn't occur to you to question them
Unhelpful: they don't lead to useful responses
Distorted: they don't fit the facts
Demoralising: they keep your mood low
Involuntary: they come to your mind automatically
Negative: they focus on the worst possible outcome
Groundless: they are usually untrue

> Distortions are good news because they mean the thoughts are probably untrue and don't need to cause you distress or keep you from managing your pain.

EXAMPLES OF NEGATIVE AUTOMATIC THOUGHTS

1. **Overgeneralisation**. You look at things in absolute, black-and-white terms. If you find yourself thinking with words such as 'everything', 'nothing', 'always', 'never', 'everyone' and 'no one', then you are probably using this distortion.

   Example: *Everything always* turns out wrong when I do it.

2. **Mental filter**. You focus on one negative detail and filter out the larger picture.

   Example: I *can't stand* for long [single detail] so I'm useless at preparing a meal [larger picture].

3. **Jumping to conclusions**. You predict that things will turn out badly with no real evidence.

   Example: If I do that again, *it will be a disaster*.

Speechmark ⑤ ℗ This page may be photocopied for instructional use only © 2014 Keren Fisher and Susan Childs

4. **Mind reading**. You assume people are reacting negatively towards you with no real evidence.

   Example: My friends didn't ring me today. *They must think I'm a nuisance.*

5. **Catastrophising**. You make the situation out to be much worse than it is.

   Example: My life with this pain is *completely ruined.*

6. **Labelling**. You label yourself with strong disapproval.

   Example: I did that wrong. *I'm such a fool. I'm useless.*

7. **Emotional reasoning**. You think something about yourself must be true because you strongly believe it.

   Example: I feel so depressed. *I must be a really miserable person.*

8. **Personalisation and blame**. You blame yourself for something you weren't entirely responsible for, or you blame others when your own approach might contribute to a problem.

   Example: *I'm such a nuisance to everyone* when I make the bus wait while I sit down, but the *driver is very rude* to me when I complain.

9. **'Should' statements**. You criticise yourself or other people with using words such as 'should' or 'shouldn't', 'must', 'ought' and 'have to'.

   Example: I *should* be able to do this. You *have to* help me more.

10. **Dual standard**. You judge yourself with harsher criticism than you would your best friends.

    Example: I'm a *really useless specimen* now that I have this pain.

SOME ALTERNATIVES TO NEGATIVE AUTOMATIC THOUGHTS

1. **Overgeneralisation**. Instead of *'Everything always turns out wrong when I do it'*, you could think:

   'Sometimes things go wrong and sometimes they don't. Most people find the same.'

2. **Mental filter**. Instead of *'I can't stand for long so I'm useless at preparing a meal'*, you could think:

   'I can't stand for long so I'll organise the cooking into small tasks and do them one at a time.'

3. **Jumping to conclusions**. Instead of *'If I do that again, it will be a disaster'*, you could think:

   'The way I set about that wasn't successful. I'll try a different approach next time.'

4. **Mind reading**. Instead of *'My friends didn't ring me today. They must think I'm a nuisance'*, you could think:

   'Perhaps something happened to one of them. I'd better check they're OK.'

5. **Catastrophising**. Instead of *'My life with this pain is completely ruined'*, you could think:

   'My life with this pain is different. I'll think of new ways to do the things I really want to do.'

6. **Labelling**. Instead of *'I did that wrong. I'm such a fool. I'm useless'*, you could think:

   'I made a mistake. I'll try again.'

7. **Emotional reasoning**. Instead of *'I feel so depressed. I must be a really miserable person'*, you could think:

   'I feel low today. I'll try to organise a pleasant activity for myself.'

8. **Personalisation and blame**. Instead of *'I'm such a nuisance to everyone when I make the bus wait while I sit down, but the driver is very rude to me when I complain'*, you could think:

   'I'll apologise in advance for being so slow. Then people will be less likely to get annoyed.'

Speechmark ⓟ This page may be photocopied for instructional use only © 2014 Keren Fisher and Susan Childs

9. **'Should' statements**. Instead of *'I should be able to do this. You have to help me more'*, you could think:

'I can't find a way to do this at the moment. Would you mind helping me?'

10. **Dual standard**. Instead of *'I'm a really useless specimen now that I have this pain'*, you could think:

'I would say to my best friend, "There's a lot you can still achieve in spite of the pain".'

A TASK FOR YOU

Try to identify the distortions in these PUDDING thoughts. Put the appropriate number(s) from the list below into the table.

1. Overgeneralisation
2. Mental filter
3. Jumping to conclusions
4. Mind reading
5. Catastrophising
6. Labelling
7. Emotional reasoning
8. Personalisation and blame
9. 'Should' statements
10. Dual standard

	Thought	Distortion(s)
1	I'm never going to succeed at this	
2	I'm so slow, I'm a real idiot	
3	If this goes on, I'll end up unable to walk	
4	Nothing I do is ever good enough now that I have this pain	
5	I'm a failure as a parent – my children are so thoughtless	
6	Since I've had this pain all I see is a lot of hopelessness	
7	My friends don't want to meet me now I've got this pain	
8	I'm a burden on everyone now	
9	I should be able to do tasks like I used to	
10	I feel so depressed, I'm useless	

Speechmark ⑤ Ⓟ This page may be photocopied for instructional use only © 2014 Keren Fisher and Susan Childs

A TASK FOR YOU

Try this exercise using an example from your own life.

Mood Log 2

You can practise recognising distortions in PUDDING thoughts by filling in this form. Jot down some more thoughts. If they are associated with unpleasant or negative emotions, try to identify whether you have used one or more negative automatic thought distortions from the list provided.

1. Overgeneralisation
2. Mental filter
3. Jumping to conclusions
4. Mind reading
5. Catastrophising
6. Labelling
7. Emotional reasoning
8. Personalisation and blame
9. 'Should' statements
10. Dual standard

Step 1: Describe the upsetting **situation or event**.

Step 2: **Feelings**. What emotion did you feel? (For example, angry, sad, anxious)
How much? (On a scale from 0 to 100 per cent)
Remember to use only one word for each feeling.

Step 3: **Thought**. What did you think at the time of this situation or event?
How true would you rate this thought? (On a scale from 0 to 100 per cent)

Step 4: **Negative interpretations**. Record the number(s) of the distorted interpretations that apply.

Speechmark ⓟ This page may be photocopied for instructional use only © 2014 Keren Fisher and Susan Childs

CHALLENGING NEGATIVE AUTOMATIC THOUGHTS

Unhelpful feelings (negative emotions) alert you to the need for catching and investigating your thoughts (cognitions). In **cognitive behavioural therapy** it's helpful to look at your *behaviour* too. This could involve **becoming your own scientist**.

One of the common ways in which thoughts are distorted is to *jump to conclusions* that things turn out badly, without giving yourself the chance to try them out.

Doing behavioural experiments

In order to test out your thoughts, imagine you are a scientist, keen to learn a response to an experiment without being able to predict the result before the task is completed.

> Experiments allow you to learn about the real outcome of a situation rather than your feared one.
>
> For example, you might think that your friends don't invite you when they meet for lunch because they find your company depressing.

Your *thought* about this situation is:

> 'They don't invite me because they will notice I have pain and it will upset them.'

Your *belief* in this thought is 95 per cent.

You sometimes have an *alternative thought*:

> 'They won't notice my pain if I join in cheerfully.'

Your *belief* in this thought is 5 per cent.

You could design an experiment to test out which thought turns out to be more realistic.

Behavioural experiments can be quite *scary* – you are putting yourself in a vulnerable position. You might find your thought was true after all. However, experiments are very useful because they are 'no fail'. Whether they work out entirely successfully or not, you gather information to help you change and to possibly try a more helpful experiment next time.

You could think that as a scientist you need to prepare for any outcome and remain *curious* about finding out more about it.

Speechmark P This page may be photocopied for instructional use only © 2014 Keren Fisher and Susan Childs

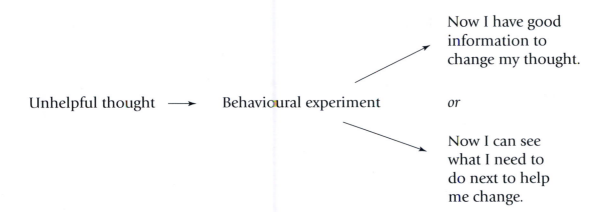

Unhelpful thought ⟶ Behavioural experiment

Now I have good information to change my thought.

or

Now I can see what I need to do next to help me change.

Behavioural experiment example

Step 1: What is the thought about this situation?
How true is it? (On a scale from 0 to 100 per cent)

'My friends don't invite me because they will notice my pain and it will upset them.'
95 per cent

Step 2: What alternative thought could you have?
How true is it? (On a scale from 0 to 100 per cent)

'They won't notice my pain if I join in cheerfully.'
5 per cent

Step 3: What experiment will help you test which thought is true?

'I will invite one or two of my best friends to join me for lunch. I will think of some amusing things to tell them. I will suggest I join in with them next week and see if they agree.'

Step 4: What was the outcome?

'My friends said they enjoyed our meeting and they want to see me again next week.'

Speechmark Ⓟ This page may be photocopied for instructional use only © 2014 Keren Fisher and Susan Childs

Step 5: How true is the thought from Step 1 now? (On a scale from 0 to 100 per cent)

20 per cent

Step 6: How true is the alternative thought from Step 2 now? (On a scale from 0 to 100 per cent)

70 per cent

Speechmark ⓅThis page may be photocopied for instructional use only © 2014 Keren Fisher and Susan Childs

A TASK FOR YOU

Try this exercise using an example from your own life. Decide on a situation or event that gives you negative emotional feelings.

> **Step 1**: What is the thought about this situation or event?
> How true is it? (On a scale from 0 to 100 per cent)

> **Step 2**: What alternative thought could you have?
> How true is it? (On a scale from 0 to 100 per cent)

> **Step 3**: What experiment will help you test which thought is true?

> **Step 4**: What was the outcome?

> **Step 5**: How true is the thought from Step 1 now? (On a scale from 0 to 100 per cent)

> **Step 6**: How true is the alternative thought from Step 2 now? (On a scale from 0 to 100 per cent)

Speechmark ⑤ Ⓟ This page may be photocopied for instructional use only © 2014 Keren Fisher and Susan Childs

WEIGHING UP THE EVIDENCE

One way of challenging negative automatic thoughts is to weigh the evidence for and against their being true. This makes it easier to see whether your negative interpretation of a situation is true or whether a more realistic one is more appropriate. Behavioural experiments are a good way for you to collect evidence.

The important point is to concentrate on the *facts* that the evidence shows you rather than opinions or interpretations. For this you could think of yourself as a judge in a court of law, examining the evidence from each side of the argument in turn and then weighing up which is the most likely verdict.

> If the evidence is mostly against the thought being true, then there is *good news*, because you don't need to hang on to negative emotions and responses. You can decide to substitute more realistic interpretations that can help you improve your life.

For example, if you can't walk upstairs but you are scared of the lifts in a place you visit often, you might think: *'The lift will get stuck and I'll be trapped for hours.'* You *believe* this is 80 per cent true and your *anxiety* is high at 85 per cent.

You could find out how often the lifts have got stuck and weigh up the evidence of your thought being true.

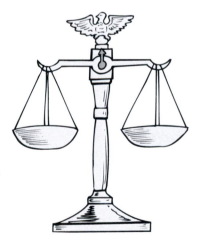

Evidence for the thought
- A lot of people avoid lifts.
- All machinery is likely to fail sometimes.
- You hear of people stuck in lifts quite often.
- These lifts look quite old.

Evidence against the thought
- They told me the lifts are well maintained.
- One lift failed two years ago but no one was trapped.
- The other lifts were all OK.
- They fixed the broken one within 20 minutes.

With this information you could substitute a *more realistic thought*:

'The lift isn't likely to trap me. They'll get me out quickly if necessary.'

- Your *belief* in your original thought is 40 per cent now.
- Your *belief* in the more realistic thought is 60 per cent.

The behavioural experiment can test it out. Try travelling one floor in the lift.

 Speechmark Ⓟ This page may be photocopied for instructional use only © 2014 Keren Fisher and Susan Childs

After your behavioural experiment:

- your *belief* in your original thought is 10 per cent
- your *belief* in the more realistic thought is 75 per cent
- your *anxiety* has reduced to 20 per cent and you feel confident to travel in the lift again.

A TASK FOR YOU

Thought-challenging worksheet

Step 1: Describe the upsetting **situation or event**.

Step 2: **Feelings**. What emotion did you feel? (For example, angry, sad, anxious)
How much? (On a scale from 0 to 100 per cent)

Step 3: **Thought**. What is the thought about this situation?
How true is it? (On a scale from 0 to 100 per cent)

Step 4: What is the **evidence** for and against the thought?

For   *Against*

_____   _____
_____   _____
_____   _____

Step 5: **Alternative interpretation**. What could be an alternative thought about the situation or event now you have the evidence?
How true is the alternative thought? (On a scale from 0 to 100 per cent)

Step 6: How true is the original thought from Step 3 now? (On a scale from 0 to 100 per cent)

Step 7: **Feelings**. How bad are your emotions from Step 2 now? (On a scale from 0 to 100 per cent)

Speechmark ⑤ ℗ This page may be photocopied for instructional use only © 2014 Keren Fisher and Susan Childs

CORE BELIEFS

Core beliefs are a particular form of automatic thoughts that are usually rigid, negative and reflect long-standing ideas about yourself and your life. They have usually been formed in childhood, possibly by a distracted parent who undermined your self-esteem. This may have led to a core belief that you are worthless and unlovable. This belief then acts as a filter or funnel through which you interpret the world around you. You take this for granted and it does not occur to you to question it.

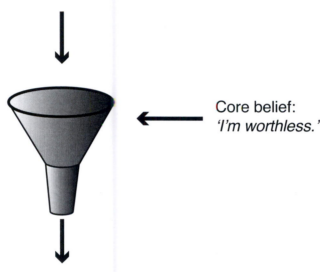

Friends say: '*You're really good company.*'

Core belief: '*I'm worthless.*'

They don't mean it.

FIGURE 4 Core belief as a funnel

Core beliefs are maintained by focusing on interpretations of events that tend to support those core beliefs and by ignoring any evidence that appears to contradict them.

You will recognise that a core belief is lurking around if you notice a mismatch between your *feelings* and your *thoughts* when you are trying to do the tasks in your therapy programme.

> For example, your emotion might be quite strong. Perhaps you rate depression at 80 per cent but when you try to identify the thought that preceded it, you come up with a trivial interpretation such as: '*I did that exercise quite slowly.*'

> There is no real reason why this thought should arouse a strong depression response, so ask yourself: '*If that thought were true, why is it a problem?*' This will produce another thought, such as: '*People will think I'm lazy.*'

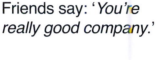

Ask yourself the question again: *'If that thought were true, why is it a problem?'* This might produce a new thought such as: *'They won't respect me.'*

Ask yourself the question again: *'If that thought were true, why is it a problem?'* A new thought might be: *'They will leave me and I shall be abandoned.'*

This seems like the core belief and fits better with a strong feeling of depression.

Core beliefs are ideas, *not facts*, and they can be challenged like any other thought, but they need to be unearthed and identified. This process will uncover other unrealistic and distorted thoughts along the way.

Speechmark Ⓟ This page may be photocopied for instructional use only © 2014 Keren Fisher and Susan Childs

A TASK FOR YOU

Use this list to identify the negative automatic distortions in the thoughts leading to the core belief. Each downward arrow means: *'If that were true, why is it a problem?'*

1. Overgeneralisation
2. Mental filter
3. Jumping to conclusions
4. Mind reading
5. Catastrophising
6. Labelling
7. Emotional reasoning
8. Personalisation and blame
9. 'Should' statements
10. Dual standard

> Situation: your physiotherapist says, *'Let's do that exercise again.'*

Thought   **Distortion(s)**

They're repeating it because I didn't do it well enough. I feel really depressed now.	
I'm not as good as the others. I'm stupid.	
People will notice I'm no good at this.	
They will avoid me.	
I will be isolated and abandoned.	
I am unlovable.	

Speechmark ℗ This page may be photocopied for instructional use only © 2014 Keren Fisher and Susan Childs

TASK

    A TASK FOR YOU

Try this exercise with an example from your own life. If you have a strong emotion that does not fit the first thought, track down to a core belief.

Use the list to identify the negative automatic distortions in the thoughts leading to the core belief. Each downward arrow means: *'If that were true, why is it a problem?'*

1. Overgeneralisation
2. Mental filter
3. Jumping to conclusions
4. Mind reading
5. Catastrophising
6. Labelling
7. Emotional reasoning
8. Personalisation and blame
9. 'Should' statements
10. Dual standard

Situation:

Feelings: What emotion did you feel?
How much? (On a scale from 0 to 100 per cent)

Thought

Distortion(s)

Speechmark P This page may be photocopied for instructional use only © 2014 Keren Fisher and Susan Childs

SUMMARY: HOW THOUGHTS INFLUENCE YOUR LIFE WITH PAIN

The following list is a summary of CBT techniques to understand how thoughts influence your life with pain and what to do about them.

1. Emotions and behavioural responses are driven by *thoughts*.
2. It is necessary to distinguish between *thoughts* and *emotions*.
3. Thoughts are *not facts*. They are interpretations based on past experience, opinions and moods.
4. Facts have evidence (things you can see, hear, touch, and so on) and can be proved.
5. Weighing up the evidence can identify where thoughts are distorted (PUDDING thoughts).
6. Behavioural experiments can supply you with the evidence you need.
7. Distorted thoughts can be challenged with the evidence.
8. Core beliefs about the self will influence how situations and events are interpreted. Beliefs can be challenged like other thoughts.
9. Identifying negative distortions and substituting more realistic thoughts supplied by the evidence will improve your unhelpful negative reactions and allow you to achieve more of the life you want.

TASK

 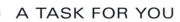 A TASK FOR YOU

Try this exercise with an example from your own life. Use this form to record how you challenge thoughts that stop you living the life you want.

Mood Log 3

Step 1: Describe the upsetting **situation or event**.

Step 2: **Feelings**. What emotion did you feel? (For example, angry, sad, anxious)
How much? (On a scale from 0 to 100 per cent)

Step 3: **Thoughts**. What did you think at the time of this situation or event?
How true would you rate these thoughts? (On a scale from 0 to 100 per cent)

Step 4: **Negative interpretations**. Record the distorted interpretations that apply.

Step 5: **Alternative responses**. What does the evidence show you?
Substitute more realistic thoughts. How true are they? (On a scale from 0 to 100 per cent)

Step 6: **Outcome**. How true are your thoughts from Step 3 now? (On a scale from 0 to 100 per cent)

Step 7: **Feelings**. How bad are your emotions from Step 2 now? (On a scale from 0 to 100 per cent)

Speechmark ⑤ ℗ This page may be photocopied for instructional use only © 2014 Keren Fisher and Susan Childs

An Introduction to Acceptance and Commitment Therapy

Acceptance and commitment therapy (ACT) has its focus on giving up the struggle to achieve some other state and instead to experience how things are at this moment in an accepting, non-judgemental fashion.

ACT involves:
- *acceptance* of some pain or discomfort that is out of your personal control
- *commitment* to taking action towards the things that are important to you (values)
- *testing out* new ways of thinking and feeling.

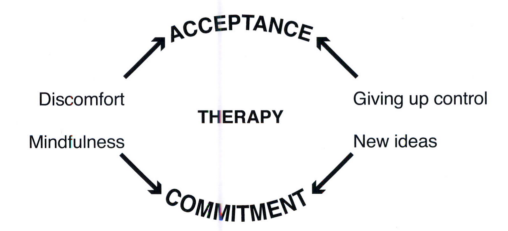

ACT has six core processes.

1. Acceptance of discomfort and painful feelings, rather than trying to get rid of them
2. Being present – being right here, right now – also called mindfulness
3. Defusing – breaking the bond between thought 'rules' and actions
4. Values – the things that really give your life meaning
5. Committed action towards values even if it involves difficult challenges
6. Spending more time with your 'observing' self – the core, unchanging you who notices passing thoughts and feelings without necessarily reacting

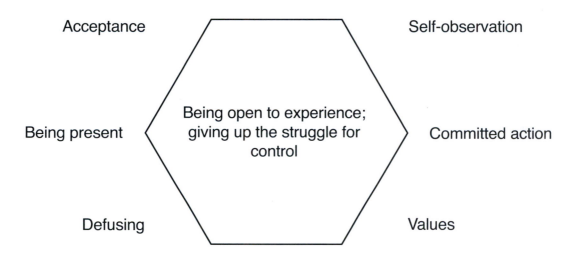

ACCEPTANCE AND COMMITMENT THERAPY: THE SIX CORE PROCESSES AS APPLIED TO PAIN

1. Acceptance involves allowing your pain sensations, thoughts and feelings to be exactly as they are without trying to change them or control them, even though they are uncomfortable. It is the *key to flexibility*.
2. Being present involves mindfulness. This means being aware of what you are experiencing right here, right now in this present moment without judging it as right or wrong, pleasant or unpleasant.
3. Defusing involves not allowing thoughts to control you. It is about detaching your thoughts from the things that you want to do but which you have been avoiding because of your pain thoughts. Thoughts are not rules. You do not have to obey them.
4. Values involve identifying the things that really matter to you more than your pain, such as improvement in relationships, work, personal development and health.
5. Committed action involves doing what it takes to move towards your values, even if it causes some discomfort.
6. Self-observation involves attending to that part of yourself that can stand back and observe all your thoughts and feelings as they pass through your mind. You notice them but are not changed by them because your 'core' self is witnessing rather than producing the thoughts.

Speechmark ⑤ Ⓟ This page may be photocopied for instructional use only © 2014 Keren Fisher and Susan Childs

1. ACCEPTANCE OR MIND PING-PONG

Acceptance is not the same as giving up hope, nor is it assuming nothing can change. It is an active process of being aware of how things are, rather than how they 'should' be.

This can be quite a difficult idea for people with long-term pain. They often struggle with thoughts about how things were in the past and what they wish for (and fear) in the future. Their thoughts sometimes oscillate back and forth between past and future like a game of mind ping-pong.

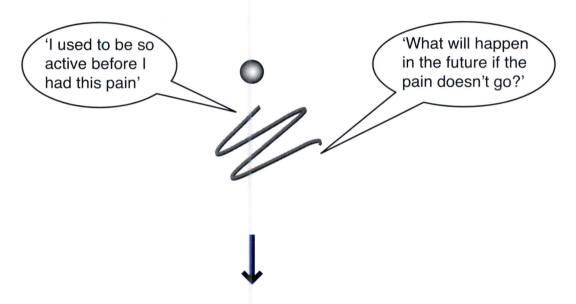

Acceptance is stopping the mind ping-pong and being willing to have pain but also to have more of the life you want. This could mean the pain becomes easier to manage in the context of a richer life.

Being flexible and prepared to move your behaviour in the direction of the things you value rather than in the direction of pain relief is the key to ACT.

It is a process you can choose to engage in.

You can choose to be willing to 'let go' of trying to control your situation and instead to experience new ways of thinking and responding.

The only outcome you're looking for from these experiences is an answer to the question:

'Do they help me move towards my valued activities?'

If the answer is *yes*, then that is what works.

A TASK FOR YOU

Thinking about acceptance, can you tell the effect these thoughts would have on moving towards your valued life direction?

Old thoughts about acceptance	Effects on action?	New thoughts about acceptance	Effects on action?
I cannot change		I can live a valued life alongside this pain	
Pain is a death sentence		I can give up the struggle but still approach my life values	
I have invested all this time trying to get better		I can stop the tug of war with my pain problem	
It is all hopeless		I do not have to think about controlling the pain; I can focus on my values instead	
I am stuck with this pain		I can concentrate on how things are, not how they were or how they might become	
There is nothing I can do		I do not have to let my thoughts dictate my actions	

Speechmark P This page may be photocopied for instructional use only © 2014 Keren Fisher and Susan Childs

Acceptance is a new way of looking at pain

Acceptance involves being willing to allow for some discomfort. It also encourages you to give up the struggle to get rid of it. Fighting with your pain wastes energy and takes time away from pursuing what is really important to you.

You will have made valiant efforts to get control of the pain and have probably invested money as well as time in the process. *This is natural. The normal response is to try to improve an unpleasant situation*, but things may not have worked out as well as you hoped.

If you think of your pain as a monster, you could imagine that you spend a lot of time and energy having a tug of war with it. If the pain wins, you will fall into a deep pit, so you try to pull the monster into the pit instead.

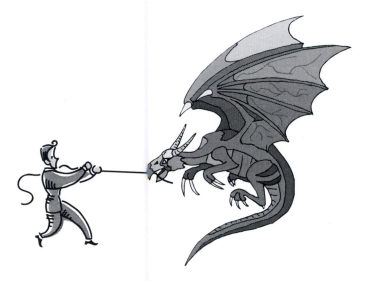

If you have been acting like this for some time, now would be a good opportunity to ask yourself:

'Has the monster got smaller? Is my pain better?'

The answer is probably *no*. All the things you have tried have only served to demonstrate that seeking to gain control is a vain hope.

Acceptance means you are willing to have the pain (as you've learned you can't make it go away), but you are progressing with more important aspects of your life alongside it.

As an alternative, you could just *let go of the rope* and attend to more valuable activities instead. The pain monster will still be around but it can't go on fighting with you, as the strong connection you had before has been loosened.

A TASK FOR YOU

List some of the things you have done to try to improve your situation.

Something you have tried	Did this help or did it make things worse?	Did this enable you to move towards your important valued activities?	Did this create energy and fitness or did it use your energy and fitness up?
1			
2			
3			
4			
5			

Speechmark P This page may be photocopied for instructional use only © 2014 Keren Fisher and Susan Childs

2. BEING PRESENT: MINDFULNESS

How can mindfulness help to manage the pain?

When you experience pain and suffering, you need to consider these questions:
- What is suffering? Is it the same as pain?
- What do you notice when you have pain?
- Does it look a bit like this?

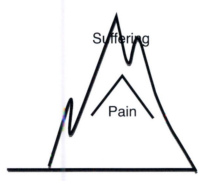

These are some typical answers that people with chronic pain give when they are asked how they experience their pain. Does this seem familiar to you?

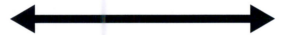

Past	Here and now	Future
I used to go to the gym twice a week but then I had pain.		I won't be able to go to the gym again – it is too painful.
I used to care for my grandchildren but then the pain got too bad.	?	My grandchildren will not need me to look after them by the time I am better.
I used to work in the charity shop but then this pain started.		I cannot imagine myself going back to work until I get rid of this pain.

The entries on this table are not about the *sensation* of pain. They are thoughts and beliefs.

Why is there nothing in the middle? Sometimes people feel as if they are trapped between thoughts and sensations from the past and worries and concerns about the future. Does this feel to you like a battle between the past and the future?

> It is this pathway from the past to the future (and back) that causes the battle and much of the suffering.

Staying in the 'here and now'

We can stop the battle by choosing to stay in the here and now no matter what we are doing or feeling.

A TASK FOR YOU

Try this experiment (this is usually done with raisins, but water might be more convenient).

Take a drink of water – just a sip. Concentrate on the sensations the water creates as it reaches your lips and then as it enters your mouth. Notice the temperature of the water – refreshing, cooling or shockingly cold. Pay attention to the sensation. Notice the muscular action of swallowing. Follow the sensations of the water passing down into your stomach. Notice the temperature change as the water warms up in your body.

Just stay with these sensations. Maybe the thoughts and emotions about suffering are still there. They may even try to bother you, but you can choose to stay with the sensations of drinking water.

Record what happened. What did your brain do? Could you stay 'in the moment' with all the other thoughts and emotions going round in your mind?

Yes, I could stay in the moment	No, I could not concentrate on the water
I could feel:	I could feel:

What does this little exercise tell you about the habits of your brain?

_____

_____

_____

_____

Speechmark P This page may be photocopied for instructional use only © 2014 Keren Fisher and Susan Childs

Ifs and buts and suffering

Coping with chronic pain can change your life so that it seems all there is left is pain and suffering. What valued activities have you given up?

Try this exercise with an example from your own life.

I used to:	*But*

Do these statements focus on *you* or the *suffering*?

Now try this: replace the *but* with *and*.

I used to:	*And*

How does it feel now? Is the focus still on the suffering?

So it looks as if pain and suffering are not the same. Practising being in the here and now with mindfulness can help you to let go of the struggle between the past and the future.

Changing your internal thoughts and your external language can help you to weaken the bond between pain and suffering so that you can choose:

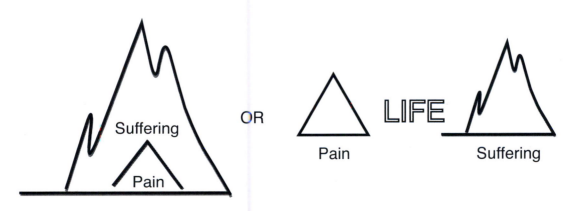

3. DEFUSION OF THOUGHTS AND ACTIONS

This is an introduction to another method of dealing with thoughts.

Our mind is a powerful machine for converting sensory experience into thought. Words transform the way we perceive things and can eventually take the place of actual experience. We do not need to be attacked by a tiger to see the connection between the words 'tiger' and 'danger'.

TIGER　　　　DANGER

The sensory experience of seeing a tiger automatically triggers a thought such as:

'This is dangerous. I must keep a safe distance to avoid getting injured.'

So, if you have experienced a situation in which your pain seemed worse, it is not necessary to experience every similar situation for your mind to produce the thought: *I must avoid doing this, as it will cause more pain.* Your mind has converted an image of the situation into a symbol for danger without your being aware of it.

DANGER

Gradually your mind (all the time trying to keep you out of danger) will convince you that many of your valued activities have the label

DANGER

and must be avoided. Your mind has created a thought about danger and you respond with the danger rule: *I must avoid doing this, as it will cause more pain.*

ACT encourages us to 'defuse' thoughts and reactions so that words lose their power to determine what we will do next. When thoughts and actions are unglued or 'defused', valued activities can continue in spite of thoughts that try to derail us.

Speechmark ⑤　ⓟ This page may be photocopied for instructional use only © 2014 Keren Fisher and Susan Childs

A TASK FOR YOU

This exercise is about recognising thought habits and their effects.

	What thought about pain did your mind produce?	What response did you make when you believed or obeyed the thought?	Was this a good or a bad outcome?
Day 1			
Day 2			
Day 3			
Day 4			
Day 5			
Day 6			
Day 7			

4. VALUES

A value is an aspect of life that really matters to you. It acts as a principle to guide your life in your desired directions.

Speechmark ℗ This page may be photocopied for instructional use only © 2014 Keren Fisher and Susan Childs

A TASK FOR YOU

Before the onset of your pain problem, what were the main values in your life?

Here are some headings to help you. Fill in any that are useful for you.

1. **Relationships with your spouse or partner** – how did you want them to be?

2. **Relationships with your children** – how did you want them to be?

3. **Employment** – what kind of work did you want to do?

4. **Personal development** – did you want to learn something new, attend classes or continue your education?

5. **Hobbies and leisure** – what did you want to do with your spare time?

6. **Working in your community** – did you want to volunteer for community projects, serve in the charity shop or something similar?

7. **Social life** – how did you want your relationships with your friends to be?

8. **Health** – how did you want to look after your physical fitness?

5. COMMITTED ACTION

Committed action is about being willing to give up avoidance of activities and to experience new things in the direction of your values.

Speechmark P This page may be photocopied for instructional use only © 2014 Keren Fisher and Susan Childs

A TASK FOR YOU

Your life with pain – what actions have you made in the last week towards your chosen values?

Fill in this form to help you focus on how you can lead your life even with your long-term pain.

Day	Day of week	What actions have you taken?
Day 1		
Day 2		
Day 3		
Day 4		
Day 5		
Day 6		
Day 7		

Speechmark P This page may be photocopied for instructional use only © 2014 Keren Fisher and Susan Childs

6. OBSERVER SELF

The observer you is your stable core, which watches your thoughts and emotions passing along as if in a stream. The stream is not changed by the thoughts. It contains them without responding to them just like your observer self contains your thoughts but remains detached and non-judgemental.

Imagine giving an account of yourself at a job interview or to someone you have just met for the first time, or to someone you have engaged in a discussion about local politics.

The *you* who is giving the accounts is your stable core that has been with you all your life, but this *you* tends to get lost in the constant busyness of your mind.

> When you first try to spend time with your observer self, you might encounter your internal critic, who reminds you of your pain and your habitual thoughts of avoidance and the loss of your valued activities.

> If you take a further step back, you can observe all these thoughts without reacting to or judging them.
>
> When you hear your internal critic, you can acknowledge it (*there goes my critic thought again*), and allow the thoughts to pass along until you can step back and observe them without judgement. *That is your observer self.*

You are the person right here, right now, who is aware of the thoughts, memories and sensations. Your observer self sees your pain and typical responses more clearly from a distance, without getting tied up in the usual spiral of judgement and emotional reaction.

You can help to stay with your observer self by remembering the SNAIL:

Stop – take a mindful breathing space
Notice when you are processing rather than observing
Attend to the present moment
Identify thoughts that hook you in
Label them to distance yourself from them.

Speechmark ⓟ This page may be photocopied for instructional use only © 2014 Keren Fisher and Susan Childs

A TASK FOR YOU

This activity is about spending time with your observer self.

Over the next week, set a short period of time (say five minutes) just noticing your thought stream. What thought habits do you notice? Do not evaluate or judge them, just notice them.

Write them down in this table.

Practice	My thoughts are:	What habits are these?
Day 1		
Day 2		
Day 3		
Day 4		
Day 5		
Day 6		
Day 7		

Speechmark Ⓟ This page may be photocopied for instructional use only © 2014 Keren Fisher and Susan Childs

More on Mindfulness

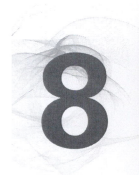

Mindfulness is not a religion!

There have been many definitions of mindfulness. It has come down to us from Eastern (mainly Buddhist) customs but has now influenced Western thought. It combines both ancient and modern meditation practices.

Everyone worries about the future and regrets things from the past – this is completely natural and sometimes your mind becomes so busy with the past and the future that it becomes unaware of the present. When you have long-term pain this is not useful, as it increases muscle tension and allows more 'danger' signals to be sent to the brain, where they are ultimately read as more pain.

> Mindfulness means paying attention to the present moment in a particular way. It is a way of *being* rather than *doing*.

- It is the opposite of being absent-minded (or being on autopilot).
- It aims to help you be in the present moment without judgement and without comparison with the past or the future.
- It helps you to allow things to be as they actually are, right here, right now, rather than reliving past failures or pre-living anticipated future failures.
- It aims to help you take control of your mind rather than allowing your mind to be in control of you.

Imagine what would happen if your mind were a puppy!
- Puppies rush about all over the place.
- They need to be trained to behave in a predictable way.
- They need consistent instructions and practice until they get the hang of what you want them to do.

Your mind is just the same.
- It needs training to keep it in check instead of rushing about with thoughts you cannot control.

Speechmark ⑤ Ⓟ This page may be photocopied for instructional use only © 2014 Keren Fisher and Susan Childs

- Your mind needs to learn to come back when you ask it to, so that it can return to the present moment. *Mindfulness exercises will help it.*

Mindfulness is not meant to:
- make you relaxed
- change things
- make you cheerful
- make you think positively.

Mindful awareness allows attention to move between the experiences of the present moment.

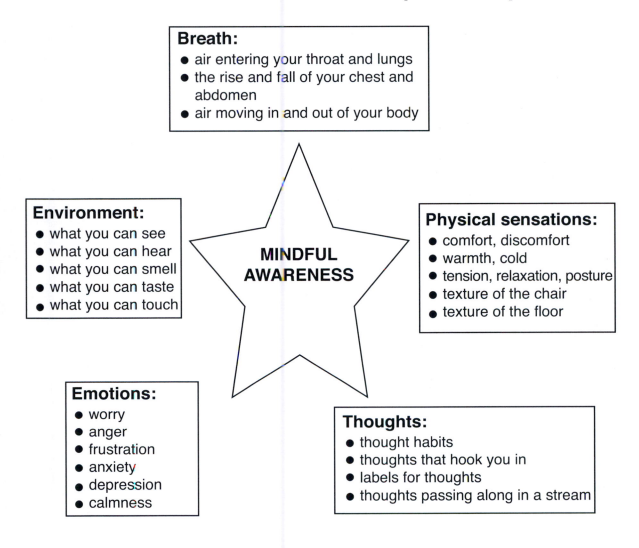

Breath:
- air entering your throat and lungs
- the rise and fall of your chest and abdomen
- air moving in and out of your body

Environment:
- what you can see
- what you can hear
- what you can smell
- what you can taste
- what you can touch

MINDFUL AWARENESS

Physical sensations:
- comfort, discomfort
- warmth, cold
- tension, relaxation, posture
- texture of the chair
- texture of the floor

Emotions:
- worry
- anger
- frustration
- anxiety
- depression
- calmness

Thoughts:
- thought habits
- thoughts that hook you in
- labels for thoughts
- thoughts passing along in a stream

MINDFUL AWARENESS OF THE BREATH

If you take a few breaths and really concentrate on the experience of the air entering and leaving your body, you are being *mindful* of the breath. While you were mindful of the sensations of breathing, your mind was not dwelling on the thoughts that lead to the downward spiral of pain and stress. Breath is often used as an anchor for mindfulness practice, as it is always available to focus attention on the present moment.

Speechmark Ⓟ This page may be photocopied for instructional use only © 2014 Keren Fisher and Susan Childs

A TASK FOR YOU: MINDFULNESS AND BREATHING

Sit up straight and keep your shoulders relaxed. Pay attention to your breathing. Notice how the breath enters your nose, throat and lungs. Follow your breath as it spreads to all areas of your body. Notice the movement of the breath in your chest and abdomen, rising and falling as the air enters and leaves. Simply pay attention to what it feels like to become aware of the full experience of breathing. Try to continue for 10 minutes or more.

When you are ready, gradually stretch your muscles and get up.

Record your experiences.

	Day 1	Day 2	Day 3	Day 4	Day 5	Day 6	Day 7
Minutes spent with this exercise							
What did you experience?							

Speechmark Ⓟ This page may be photocopied for instructional use only © 2014 Keren Fisher and Susan Childs

Mindfulness can help you tolerate physical symptoms

Sensations are in the body all the time but sometimes they get more intense and take over your consciousness so you can't concentrate properly on anything else. The more we try to control the problem the more we risk *increasing* sensations of tension, fatigue and pain. Muscles tighten and pain becomes more intense as we make stronger and stronger attempts to get control.

But time spent in trying to control sensations = less time for valued activity.

If in the past you tried to reduce your pain sensations but were unsuccessful, especially if you noticed that they became even more intrusive, you may now have developed a *phobia* that prevents you trying again. It is easy to see how this cycle can develop.

PHOBIA = Event + pain + thoughts +avoidance + fear.

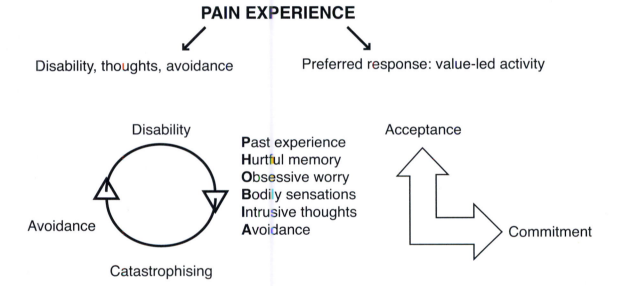

PAIN EXPERIENCE

Disability, thoughts, avoidance

Preferred response: value-led activity

Disability

Avoidance

Catastrophising

Past experience
Hurtful memory
Obsessive worry
Bodily sensations
Intrusive thoughts
Avoidance

Acceptance

Commitment

FIGURE 1 PHOBIA

Mindfulness is a good technique for desensitising a phobia about experiencing pain.

MINDFULNESS OF PHYSICAL SENSATIONS

We can begin to notice changes in the sensations associated with pain. Maybe they come in waves with episodes of relative relief between them. Perhaps there are changes in temperature. Characteristics such as *stabbing* and *tingling* might come and go. Examining the sensations like a curious scientist would allow us to observe their fluctuating nature and lets us recognise that our responses can change too.

Speechmark P This page may be photocopied for instructional use only © 2014 Keren Fisher and Susan Childs

A TASK FOR YOU: MINDFULNESS AND SENSATIONS

Sit up straight and pay attention to your breathing. Now notice what your body feels like while it is sitting on the chair with your feet on the floor. Allow your feelings to be exactly as they are in this minute. You may notice feelings of discomfort or relaxation or tension, calm or anxiety. Do not try to change them or control them. Just refocus your attention on your breath. Notice the feelings, whether pleasant and calm or unpleasant and painful. Can you describe what is going on in your body? Just notice the sensations. Try to continue for 10 minutes or more.

When you are ready, bring your attention back to your breath. Take three or four mindful breaths, then gradually stretch your muscles and get up.

Record your experiences.

	Day 1	Day 2	Day 3	Day 4	Day 5	Day 6	Day 7
Minutes spent with this exercise							
What did you experience?							

Speechmark Ⓟ This page may be photocopied for instructional use only © 2014 Keren Fisher and Susan Childs

MINDFUL AWARENESS OF THOUGHTS

Bodily discomfort has four parts:

1. the unpleasant physical sensations
2. the thoughts that are triggered by the sensations
3. the emotional reaction to the thoughts
4. the behavioural response to the thoughts and emotional reaction.

Parts 2 and 3 are the mental response to the physical symptoms.

Your mind is always busy. If you have pain, your mind is usually busy with thoughts and feelings that keep you hooked into the symptoms and the struggles you have in order to try and control or avoid pain. This gets in the way of moving towards your chosen *values*.

We can identify and label our thought processes. For example:

'That's the fear thought that stops me going out.'

Learning to label thoughts allows us to create a distance between the thought and the usual reaction.

If we can identify the thoughts we can choose how we respond to them. We can examine our thoughts and decide whether to believe them, to let them bully us and stop us getting on with our lives, or to accept them as events in the mind and to continue on our value-led journey.

You can make a choice: stay listening to your thoughts or pack them up and take them with you as you move towards your valued activities.

Mindfulness can allow you to experience yourself as the person observing your thoughts – the 'witness you' – rather than yourself as the helpless victim of your thoughts. It encourages you to suspend the habit of evaluating and judging yourself with the old familiar automatic thought processes and emotional reactions.

If you can become aware of yourself as your observer self, you will notice you can watch your thoughts but you stay untouched by their content. The 'observer you' is your stable core, which watches the passing flow of thoughts and emotions. You notice them but are not changed by them because your 'core' self is the listener rather than the speaker of the thoughts. Your core self might be like a chessboard. There are white pieces (good thoughts and feelings) and black pieces (bad thoughts and feelings). Life is a continuous battle to try to move the black pieces off the board, but the board itself is not part of the struggle. The board is your observer self, who stands back and notices the thought procession but is not changed by it.

> Mindfulness helps you become aware of the procession of your thoughts so that you can notice how they arise and pass through your mind. *Thoughts are not facts.* They are events in the mind, each one moving along and giving way to the next.

TASK

   A TASK FOR YOU: MINDFULNESS AND THOUGHTS

Pay attention to any thoughts that pop up. Notice how thoughts pass through your mind as you are trying to keep your awareness on your breath. Thoughts will try to grab your attention and tell you things that you 'should' be doing. Just let them chatter to themselves while you keep escorting your attention back to your breath. Thoughts will pass through your mind like cars on a motorway. They will distract you. Thoughts are not rules. You don't have to obey them. Label thoughts as if they were old friends – *'hello, there's my "you're no good at this" thought again'*. Let them pass along. Try to continue for 10 minutes or more.

When you are ready, bring your attention back to your breath. Take three or four mindful breaths, then gradually stretch your muscles and get up.

Record your experiences.

	Day 1	Day 2	Day 3	Day 4	Day 5	Day 6	Day 7
Minutes spent with this exercise							
What did you experience?							

Speechmark P This page may be photocopied for instructional use only © 2014 Keren Fisher and Susan Childs

MINDFUL AWARENESS OF EMOTIONS

Mindfulness can help you tolerate emotional reactions and worry. We all worry about various aspects of life, but it often just compounds the problem we had in the first place. Worry gets us nowhere and wastes our time.

> Worry about pain makes you tense. Tension increases the amount of activity in the nervous system. Increased activity in the nervous system leads to heightened sensitivity to all kinds of other sensations. This is all bad news and leads to increasingly negative outcomes, including increased pain.

> Imagine your worry about your pain is a loose thread in your jumper. You *work at your worry* like you might pull the loose thread. The worry becomes the main focus of your activity.
>
> What happens? Does the jumper improve?
>
> It is more likely that the whole garment is destroyed. Is this a *workable* solution to your pain problem? Does your life improve or get worse?

What makes it difficult to manage your worries about pain? What is in the 'worry bag'?

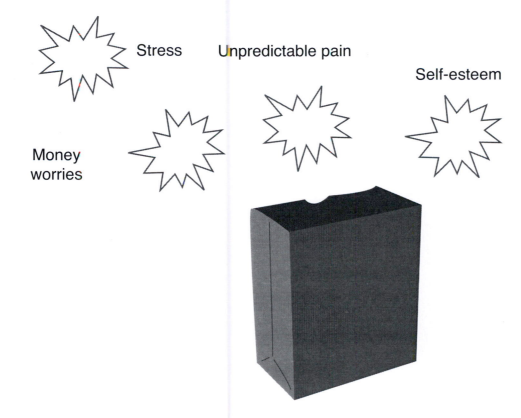

Stress   Unpredictable pain

Self-esteem

Money worries

TASK

  A TASK FOR YOU

Complete your own worry bag. What does yours contain?

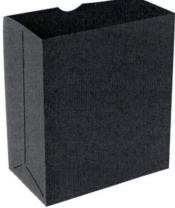

Speechmark **P** This page may be photocopied for instructional use only © 2014 Keren Fisher and Susan Childs

A TASK FOR YOU: MINDFULNESS AND EMOTIONS

Pay attention to any emotional feelings that pull you away from focusing on your breath. Do they feel good or bad, pleasant or unpleasant? Can you recognise or label a particular emotion? Let it run its natural course, rising and falling, sometimes recurring but eventually flowing away. Let yourself be with it. Take an interest in how it feels in your body without getting entangled with your usual response to it. You don't have to react, just let it flow through and subside. Try to continue for 10 minutes or more.

When you are ready, bring your attention back to your breath. Take three or four mindful breaths, then gradually stretch your muscles and get up.

Record your experiences.

	Day 1	Day 2	Day 3	Day 4	Day 5	Day 6	Day 7
Minutes spent with this exercise							
What did you experience?							

Speechmark P This page may be photocopied for instructional use only © 2014 Keren Fisher and Susan Childs

MINDFUL AWARENESS OF YOUR ENVIRONMENT

The outside world produces all sorts of stimuli to distract us. Maybe your neighbour's music, or children playing in the road, or the smell of dinner cooking disturb you when you are trying to concentrate on mindful breathing. You can let your awareness expand to create space for these experiences with a mindful approach, being open and noticing them as part of the present moment. There's no need to change anything, just accept what is present in the moment and pay attention to the outside stimuli without judging them as good or bad.

Speechmark P This page may be photocopied for instructional use only © 2014 Keren Fisher and Susan Childs

A TASK FOR YOU: MINDFULNESS AND YOUR ENVIRONMENT

Pay attention to the sounds in the room around you – concentrate on what you can hear. Don't try to identify the source of the sound, just experience it. Observe its quality, volume and pitch. If there are no sounds, just notice the silence.

Keep your eyes open and notice anything you can see in the room around you. Focus on one particular object and notice what happens if you keep your eyes still.

Notice any taste in your mouth or smell in your nose. Don't try to identify what it is, just experience the sensation.

Experience where your hands are and what they are touching. If they're in contact with your clothes, notice the feel of the fabric – rough or smooth, silky or heavy.

Try to continue for 10 minutes or more.

When you are ready, bring your attention back to your breath. Take three or four mindful breaths, then gradually stretch your muscles and get up.

Record your experiences.

	Day 1	Day 2	Day 3	Day 4	Day 5	Day 6	Day 7
Minutes spent with this exercise							
What did you experience?							

Speechmark ⑤ ℗ This page may be photocopied for instructional use only © 2014 Keren Fisher and Susan Childs

WISE MIND

According to the mindfulness tradition, there are three possible states of mind.

1. *The Reasonable Mind* approaches situations logically and attempts to solve problems by attending to facts.

2. *The Emotional Mind* approaches situations impulsively and responds without attending to logic or facts but with the strength of the emotional feeling at the time.

3. *The Wise Mind* provides the overlap between the two states. When attempting to solve problems, it uses *intuition*. It attends to the facts but also allows for emotional input. It produces solutions that 'feel' just right for the current situation.

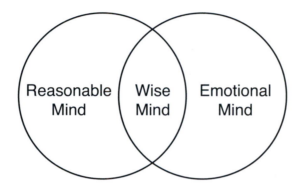

Consider the example of exercising to get fitter.

Your Reasonable Mind might say:
'Exercise has to be done every day to be of benefit.'

Your Emotional Mind might say:
'I won't do exercise. It's too painful. It makes me depressed.'

Your Wise Mind might say:
'Gently does it. It's good for you, but you need to feel rewarded for your effort. Starting small and increasing slowly won't be too hard and it will make you feel better.'

Speechmark ⓟ This page may be photocopied for instructional use only © 2014 Keren Fisher and Susan Childs

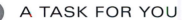 A TASK FOR YOU

Complete these boxes, using the examples to help you.

Thinking about your thoughts

Your Reasonable Mind might say:
'Thoughts are there to make plans to improve the future.'

Your Emotional Mind might say:
'My thoughts make me feel bad. They remind me how hopeless the future is likely to be and how powerless I am to change it.'

Your Wise Mind might say:
'There's no need to fix anything. Thoughts do not represent the whole truth about you or your future.'

Try an example from your own life. What does your mind say about your thoughts?
My Reasonable Mind says:

My Emotional Mind says:

My Wise Mind says:

Problem solving

Your Reasonable Mind might say:
'This situation needs a proper solution. Do whatever is necessary to find an answer.'

Your Emotional Mind might say:
'This situation is terrible. I can't concentrate on anything else. It has to improve.'

Your Wise Mind might say:
'Stand back to see what it looks like to see the problem without reacting.'

Speechmark ⑤ Ⓟ This page may be photocopied for instructional use only © 2014 Keren Fisher and Susan Childs

99

Try an example from your own life. What does your mind say about your problem situation?
My Reasonable Mind says:

My Emotional Mind says:

My Wise Mind says:

Helping friends and family

Your Reasonable Mind might say:
'Life is better if people help one another. If you make an effort you could be helpful.'

Your Emotional Mind might say:
'Since I've had this pain, I'm no use to my friends or family.'

Your Wise Mind might say:
'Acknowledge the judgements for what they are – mental events.'

Try an example from your own life. What does your mind say about helping your friends or family?
My Reasonable Mind says:

My Emotional Mind says:

My Wise Mind says:

Speechmark P This page may be photocopied for instructional use only © 2014 Keren Fisher and Susan Childs

ANOTHER USE FOR MINDFULNESS: MINDFUL EATING

People quite often eat without paying attention, possibly watching television at the same time. They do not allow themselves to savour the food or to notice the different textures or flavours. They don't notice the sensations of fullness in the stomach, so they feel unsatisfied and eat more. Or they associate watching television with eating automatically. This is a high-speed route to weight gain. Mindful eating can help you change this.

A TASK FOR YOU

The next time you have dinner, put all the foods that make up one course of your meal on a plate and sit at the table. Turn the television *off*.

Look at your food. Notice the colours, texture and patterns they make on the plate.

Spend a moment to decide which ingredient to start with. Ask yourself why you chose that particular one.

Bring the food towards your mouth, but stop to smell it first. Notice the aroma. Is it sharp? savoury? sweet? spicy?

Put it in your mouth and notice the initial taste. How would you label that?

Chew slowly attending to the flavours as they develop. Notice the change in the texture of the food and its sensations in your mouth.

Swallow and attend to the sensations of the food passing into your stomach.

Repeat this sequence for each mouthful.

What did you notice?

_____

_____

_____

_____

Speechmark ⓟ This page may be photocopied for instructional use only © 2014 Keren Fisher and Susan Childs

MINDFULNESS HELPS YOU MANAGE YOUR PAIN

As you become more practised at being a better *observer* of your thoughts, sensations and feelings, you can become more accepting of your circumstances rather than continuing the struggle to change them. By now you will have learned that this is a waste of energy. Instead, even the most distressing interpretations of your situation can be viewed from a wider perspective as passing events in the mind.

Thoughts can be viewed like conveyor belt sushi, passing along in front of you. There may be a particular thought-dish that always stops right by you. You don't specially want that thought-dish but you can't make it pass on. This is a 'sticky' thought and may need to be challenged with CBT techniques, so the conveyor belt can get 'unstuck' and move on.

POINTS TO REMEMBER

- Thoughts are not facts.
- Thoughts are just events in the mind, passing along and giving way to the next.
- You do not have to act on your thoughts. You can let them pass along like leaves in a stream, or clouds in the sky, or cars on a motorway.
- Emotions respond to thoughts. They will rise and fall like waves in the sea, each one subsiding and giving way to the next.
- You do not have to react to your emotions. You can observe them flowing through and eventually disappearing.

Memo	
1	I have pain but I am not my pain.
2	I have thoughts but I am not my thoughts.
3	I have emotions but I am not my emotions.

If you feel overwhelmed, take a breathing space. Remember the *Breath of Life*.

Breathe mindfully
Refocus attention on the present moment
Experience the movement of the breath in the body
Attend to the thoughts that come up
Think: 'thoughts are not facts but events in the mind'
Hold your attention on your breath
Escort your mind back as often as you need to

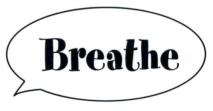

Speechmark P This page may be photocopied for instructional use only © 2014 Keren Fisher and Susan Childs

Goals and Values

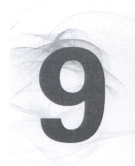

A value is an aspect of life that really matters to you. It allows you to notice whether your life at present is taking you in directions that are consistent with your personal development, or whether you are stuck in the struggle to control your pain problem and have lost sight of your ideals. Goals are helpful in deciding on activities that move you in a value-led direction.

Graded	Very important to you
Observable	Achievement oriented
Achievable	Long term
Limited	Unfinished
Specific	Encouraging
	Stimulating

Goals are different from values. A goal is a specific event, which has an end point once you have reached it. Examples of goals might be walking as far as the shops, or riding your bicycle to the local park, or losing 2 kilograms in weight.

Weight chart	
Day	**Weight**
1	85kg
2	86kg
3	87kg
4	!

By contrast, a value has no definite end point and cannot be fully achieved. It acts as a principle to guide your life in your desired direction like a compass.

Speechmark P This page may be photocopied for instructional use only © 2014 Keren Fisher and Susan Childs

You might want to be:
- a better parent
- more satisfied at work
- more economical with natural resources.

These things can't be specifically measured and they can't be completed, as they are always developing. How they progress depends on where your actions, or 'footsteps', have taken you.

> A good wedding is a goal (a completed event) but a good marriage is a value (an ongoing life-enhancing principle).

> Goal = a specific event and end point
> Value = general life direction, like a compass

VALUES AND HOW TO ACHIEVE THEM

Acceptance and commitment therapy (ACT) has some particular suggestions for values, and your job is to choose how important each one is in your life and then to think about how well you think you can succeed in moving towards that value.

ACT values could be:
- the relationship with your spouse or partner
- relationships with your children
- employment
- skills and personal development
- hobbies and leisure
- working in your community
- social life – relationships with friends
- health and fitness.

There may be several others that are particularly significant for you. It is helpful to keep a record of how much your footsteps have lead you in the direction of each of your chosen values each week.

People with chronic (long-term) health problems such as pain have often forgotten about their life values while they spend their energy seeking a cure or relief from their suffering.

ACT has its focus on giving up the struggle to achieve some other state and instead to experience how things are at this moment in an accepting, non-judgemental fashion.

It involves committing yourself to accepting some discomfort in order to achieve your goals and develop your life in a more value-led direction.

To be able to choose activities that move you towards rather than away from your values, you need to ask yourself the following questions.

'What do I want?' (that's the value)
'How do I go about it?' (that's the goal)
'What is it that is stopping me?' (that's the barrier)

IT IS USEFUL TO HAVE GOALS THAT WILL HELP YOU MOVE IN YOUR VALUE-LED DIRECTION

For example, you may decide on a value to use your leisure time better. This may involve a short-term goal such as visiting the library to get information and make notes about local activities. In this case, going to the library is a specific goal in the direction of a life value.

- Goals are actions on the way to values. They are specific things you want to achieve by a certain time.
- They allow value areas to be broken down into manageable tasks.
- They allow you to take control of your actions – rather than letting pain dictate them.
- They increase self-esteem by showing you that some important activities that you thought you would have to give up are still possible.
- They allow you to measure how much to achieve each day or week, so you get immediate feedback.

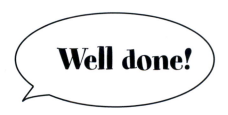

The golden rule for successful goal achievement is to make sure your goals are SMART:

Specific – so you can have a clear focus, define your activity
Measurable – so you can identify the amount you can succeed at
Achievable – so you can prioritise what is important, given other demands
Realistic – so you can make it appropriate to your lifestyle, age and ability
Timed – so you can plan how much you can progress in the time available.

Speechmark P This page may be photocopied for instructional use only © 2014 Keren Fisher and Susan Childs

A TASK FOR YOU

Having problems thinking about what goals you want to set? Check out this goal generator for some inspiration.

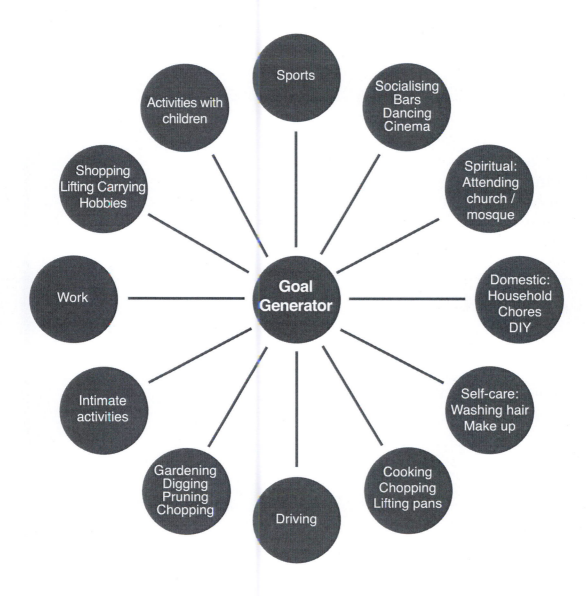

Speechmark Ⓢ Ⓟ This page may be photocopied for instructional use only © 2014 Keren Fisher and Susan Childs

TASK

     A TASK FOR YOU

Choose a value area that is important to you. Then choose goals that will help you move in the direction of that value.

My value is:

Make sure your goals are:
- Specific
- Measurable
- Achievable
- Realistic
- Timed.

My goals are:

Where am I now with this goal?

```
0    1    2    3    4    5    6    7    8    9    10
```

I have not
achieved
this goal

I have
achieved
this goal

Where am I now with this goal?

```
0    1    2    3    4    5    6    7    8    9    10
```

I have not
achieved
this goal

I have
achieved
this goal

Speechmark P This page may be photocopied for instructional use only © 2014 Keren Fisher and Susan Childs

An example

Mary wanted to improve on her social relationships value. She decided on a goal to increase her walking distance so that she could get to the coffee shop where her friends all met one morning a week. She practised walking a bit further each day to see if by the end of the week she could join her friends at their next meeting.

A goal sheet like this can help you keep a record of your success and point to possible reasons why it did or did not work out.

My goal is:	At present I can:	By next week I expect to:	Did I achieve my goal?
To have coffee with my friends in the coffee shop in town	Walk halfway to the coffee shop	Walk all the way to the coffee shop	Yes → Better than I thought → a lot [ ] / a little [ ] Yes → About what I thought [ ] No → I attempted it but missed by → a lot [ ] / a little [ ] No → I didn't attempt it [ ]

My value is better social relationships.

Mary didn't quite manage to complete her goal in the first week, so she needed to look at the *barriers* that prevented her.

Speechmark ⓢ ⓟ This page may be photocopied for instructional use only © 2014 Keren Fisher and Susan Childs

BARRIERS TO PROGRESS

There are many different kinds of barriers. Some are **physical**:

- lack of time
- lack of money
- lack of opportunity.

Others are **environmental**:

- unsuitable weather
- inaccessible buildings
- too great a distance.

There are often **internal** barriers as well:

- anxiety
- worry
- pain
- negative thoughts.

All these barriers need to be considered when you are intending to move your life in a value-led direction. They usually contain the word **but**.

Your instructions to yourself might look like this:

> I want to reach my goal *but*
> I have pain /I don't feel like it today /I don't think I can succeed at it.

It's important to recognise the type of **BUT Barrier** you are using and then think of a way to get round it.

In ACT, the most important question to ask yourself is:

> 'Do my footsteps or actions take me in the direction of my value if I listen to the advice of my thoughts and feelings?'

If the answer is *no*, try thinking of some solutions.

Thoughts as spectacles

Barriers are thoughts, but *thoughts are not facts*. Words are not rules, however much they seem to be. Barriers can be considered as just words, not whether they are true or false. Some therapists say:

> 'You can look at your values through your thoughts as if they were spectacles.'

Speechmark ⓟ This page may be photocopied for instructional use only © 2014 Keren Fisher and Susan Childs

This means you might evaluate your direction as too difficult because the view through the barriers is too indistinct.

Alternatively, you can look at your values *with* the thoughts and take them along with you on your value-led journey.

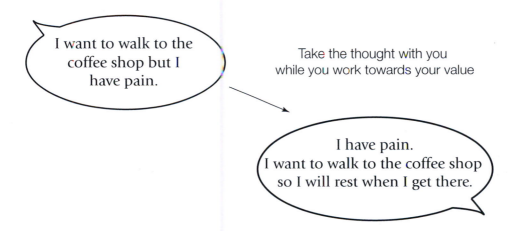

DEALING WITH BARRIERS

With any barrier (physical, environmental or internal), a step on the way to finding a solution is to remember the four Ps rule.

Problem solving   Prioritising   Planning   Pacing

ACTION PLAN

What	When	Where	How

- Problem solving = instead of thinking, *'I can't do that'*, it involves identifying where the problem lies and asking yourself, *'What is it that is stopping me achieve this task?'* Then it may be possible to look for possible solutions – for example, use a different tool or route or position, or ask someone to help.
- Prioritising = asking yourself, *'How important is it that I do this today? Does it matter if I do it later?' 'Can some one else do this while I get on with that?'*
- Planning = *'I need to do this task in the mornings before I get too tired.' 'I shall do this on Thursday when I can rest before and after.'*
- Pacing = doing a pre-decided amount of a task at a time and then stopping (a target). In this way you can gradually increase the size of your target by adding a small *manageable* amount at a time *and sticking to it*. You need to do less than you think you can on a good pain day or you run the risk of having to rest more the next day and the next day as well – the dreaded roller-coaster approach to task (non)achievement.

Speechmark Ⓟ This page may be photocopied for instructional use only © 2014 Keren Fisher and Susan Childs

Beware the roller coaster

Roller coasters happen when you overdo a task and have a pain flare-up. Then you might not be able to go back to that task for several days. When you do attempt it again, you are fearful of more pain so you do less than before, but because you have been resting, your body complains sooner. Gradually, you think you have to give up that task completely. The result might be a downward pathway to despondency.

Speechmark Ⓟ This page may be photocopied for instructional use only © 2014 Keren Fisher and Susan Childs

A TASK FOR YOU

Complete this form for important activities in your life. First, make a guess about how much of each of your chosen activities you think you can do.

Then measure in minutes and seconds exactly what you can do of those activities on a good pain day. Repeat by measuring your times on a bad pain day and on an average pain day. Look at your timings on the form and see how far out your guesstimates were. It is likely that you overestimated what you could do on a good pain day and hence might have increased your pain level.

Accurate measurements will help you to be more aware of your precise limits in behaviours such as walking, standing, sitting, lying or perching. This will make your pacing targets easier to manage.

Activity	Guesstimate: What do I think I am able to do?	How long could I do this activity on a good pain day? (minutes)	How long could I do this activity on a bad pain day? (minutes)	How long could I do this activity on an average pain day? (minutes)	Is there a difference between my guesstimate and my actual times?

This page may be photocopied for instructional use only © 2014 Keren Fisher and Susan Childs

Speechmark

WORKING OUT YOUR PACING BASELINE AND TARGETS

Your tolerance is the time it takes for you to experience increased pain when doing an activity. Your pacing targets need to start from a realistic baseline, which can be calculated like this.

- Time yourself performing an activity (e.g. walking)
- Record in minutes and seconds when you begin to notice your pain increases from your usual level (or starts)
- Repeat the timing on three separate days, which might include a good day, an average day and a bad day
- Calculate your average time (Time 1 + Time 2 + Time 3 = total; then divide total by three).
- Take away 20 per cent from your average time to find out how long you can do an activity without it increasing your pain. This is your *pacing baseline*.
- Start to increase your *targets* by 10 per cent a week from your baseline. If that increases your pain too quickly, drop back to 5 per cent.

Here is an example.

Activity	Time 1 (good day)	Time 2 (average day)	Time 3 (bad day)	Total	Average	Take away 20 per cent	*Pacing baseline*	Add 10 per cent for each weekly target
Walking	20 minutes	11 minutes	8 minutes	39 minutes	13 minutes	−3 minutes (approx.)	10 minutes	1 minute
New walking target, Week 1	11 minutes	11 minutes	11 minutes					
Week 2	12 minutes	12 minutes	12 minutes					

By dropping back to 11 minutes on a good day, you are more likely to achieve this on a bad day, as you won't be as tired as if you had overachieved when you felt better. Gradually pacing up means you are more able to keep a consistent level of improvement.

BE PATIENT

Speechmark ⑤ Ⓟ This page may be photocopied for instructional use only © 2014 Keren Fisher and Susan Childs

A TASK FOR YOU

Try this exercise using an example from your own life.
- Time yourself performing an activity (e.g. walking)
- Record in minutes and seconds when you begin to notice your pain increases from your usual level (or starts)
- Repeat the timing on three separate days, which might include a good day, an average day and a bad day
- Calculate your average time (Time 1 + Time 2 + Time 3 = total; then divide total by three).
- Take away 20 per cent from your average time to find out how long you can do an activity without it increasing your pain. This is your *pacing baseline*.
- Start to increase your *targets* by 10 per cent a week from your baseline. If that increases your pain too quickly, drop back to 5 per cent.

Activity	Time 1 (good day)	Time 2 (average day)	Time 3 (bad day)	Average	Take away 20 per cent	Baseline	Add 10 per cent
New Target, week 1							
Week 2							
Week 3							
Week 4							
Week 5							
etc							

Speechmark Ⓟ This page may be photocopied for instructional use only © 2014 Keren Fisher and Susan Childs

LOOKING AT BARRIERS IN MORE DETAIL

Some common problems faced by people with long-term pain are:

- *I want to go to college BUT I can't afford the course* (a physical barrier).
- *I want to go swimming BUT the pool is a long way away* (an environmental barrier).
- *I want a romantic evening with my partner BUT I'm afraid my pain will stop us enjoying ourselves* (an internal thought barrier).
- *I want to go to the cinema BUT I can't sit for long in those seats* (a physical and an internal barrier).

You need to get rid of the BUTs.

Solutions might involve *prioritising* (money, energy, opportunity), *planning* (how to get a student loan, how to get to the pool, how to get agreement with your partner, choosing a seat where you can stand sometimes), *pacing* (gradually walking further, trying different intimate activities, gradually sitting for longer).

There are other ways you could reach a solution as well.

> You might think of cognitive behavioural therapy solutions such as *challenging* the barrier – what is the evidence the pool is too far, or that my pain will ruin the evening, or that I can't sit long enough? Are these *facts* or my *evaluation*? Is there an alternative interpretation of this problem that I could use?

or

> You might think of ACT solutions, such as *accepting* some discomfort in order to move in the direction of your chosen life value.

or

> You might choose a mindfulness solution: *'I will concentrate on what I'm doing right here, right now, rather than listening to the advice of my thoughts and feelings, which are telling me not to try because I won't succeed.'*

Speechmark P This page may be photocopied for instructional use only © 2014 Keren Fisher and Susan Childs

A TASK FOR YOU

Use an example from your own life for this exercise.

Decide on the value area you want to progress with. Then fill in the goal you want to work on. After a week, tick the square to indicate how successful you have been.

> My value is:

My goal is:	At present I can:	By next week I expect to:	Did I achieve my goal? Put a tick in the square on the right
			Yes — Better than I thought — a lot [ ] / a little [ ] About what I thought [ ] No — I attempted it but missed by — a lot [ ] / a little [ ] I didn't attempt it [ ]

FINDING SOLUTIONS

Mary didn't quite meet her goal of walking to the coffee shop, so she didn't think she had moved far in the direction of her social relationships value. She considered the barriers and possible solutions.

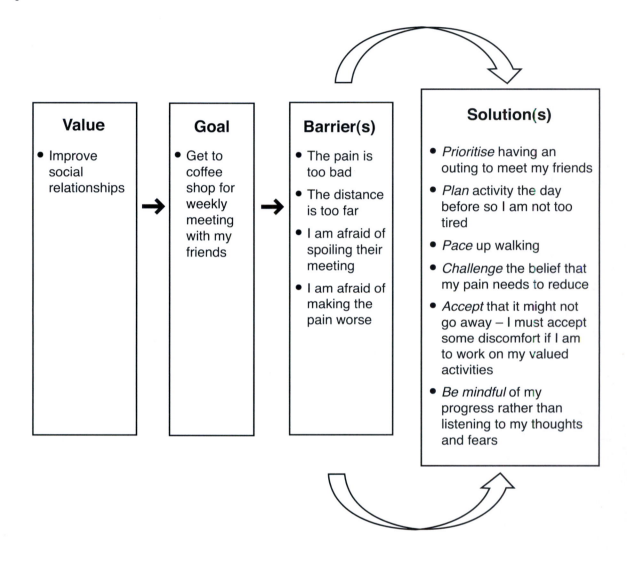

Value

- Improve social relationships

Goal

- Get to coffee shop for weekly meeting with my friends

Barrier(s)

- The pain is too bad
- The distance is too far
- I am afraid of spoiling their meeting
- I am afraid of making the pain worse

Solution(s)

- *Prioritise* having an outing to meet my friends
- *Plan* activity the day before so I am not too tired
- *Pace* up walking
- *Challenge* the belief that my pain needs to reduce
- *Accept* that it might not go away – I must accept some discomfort if I am to work on my valued activities
- *Be mindful* of my progress rather than listening to my thoughts and fears

Speechmark P This page may be photocopied for instructional use only © 2014 Keren Fisher and Susan Childs

A TASK FOR YOU

Try this exercise with an example from your own life.

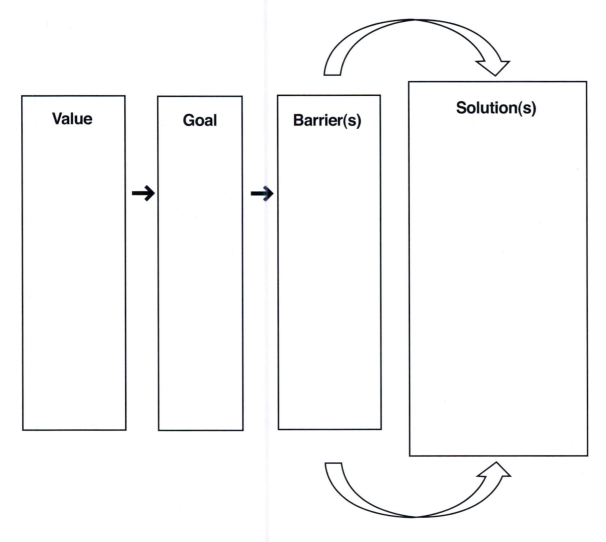

Decide which solution(s) would be best for your particular situation.

- Prioritising?
- Planning?
- Pacing?
- Cognitive behavioural therapy?
- ACT?
- Mindfulness?

A TASK FOR YOU

Keep a record of how well you have moved in your value-led direction.

Weekly value tracking sheet

Date: ………………

Value
Importance   /10

9
8
7
6
5
4
3
2
1

Value
Importance   /10

9
8
7
6
5
4
3
2
1

Value
Importance   /10

9
8
7
6
5
4
3
2
1

Value
Importance   /10

9
8
7
6
5
4
3
2
1

STEPS TOWARDS
THIS VALUE

1
2
3
4
5
6
7
8
9

Value
Importance   /10

9
8
7
6
5
4
3
2
1

Value
Importance   /10

9
8
7
6
5
4
3
2
1

Value
Importance   /10

Value
Importance   /10

9
8
7
6
5
4
3
2
1

Speechmark ⑤ Ⓟ This page may be photocopied for instructional use only © 2014 Keren Fisher and Susan Childs

More on Cognitive Defusion

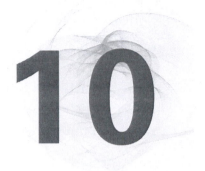

In our culture, language has a very powerful place in forming our thoughts and behaviours. For example, we can have one bad pain experience in the supermarket and then create the thought:

'Supermarkets make pain worse and should be avoided.'

The thought will then function as a barrier to undertaking activities such as shopping. We tend to follow our verbal rules even when our experience shows us that the rules don't work. A thought such as

'I will avoid doing the shopping and then my pain will get better'

encourages us to avoid shopping even though over time we notice the pain hasn't got better.

> I have pain so I will avoid doing the shopping and then my pain will get better.

> I avoided the shopping but my pain hasn't improved.

Nevertheless, we still continue to allow the thought to prevent us reaching our value-led goals because words carry meanings that spread beyond our current experience. In this example, **avoid**, **shopping** and **pain** have been fused together to form a rule that has persisted even when the evidence points in the opposite direction.

Speechmark Ⓟ This page may be photocopied for instructional use only © 2014 Keren Fisher and Susan Childs

> Acceptance and commitment therapy encourages us to unglue or *defuse* our thoughts from our reactions. 'Defusing' thoughts means valued activities can continue alongside the thought process that previously prevented forward steps in our preferred directions.

DECREASING THE HYPNOTIC POWER OF WORDS

We often behave as if our thoughts 'hypnotise' us – they make us obey them, as if we had no power to resist them.

The trick is to decrease this power and to regain our ability to make our own choices.

You could look at your thoughts and decide if they are really *believable* when they are compared with your actual experience. You can also decide if they are really *useful* in helping you on your value-led journey.

Thoughts are not rules – they are made up of words that have been collected together. You don't have to believe them.

However, you cannot *not* have them. Have you ever tried *not* thinking of a giraffe? You didn't think of it until it was put into your mind. Now you can't 'unthink' it.

Thought rules are like that. You can't make them go away. They are like fish hooks – the more you try to get free of them, the deeper they sink into you and influence your reactions.

> Thoughts can hook you in and make you believe them, but you can distance yourself from them.

There are quite a few techniques to encourage the process of distancing, ungluing or defusing words from actions.

Defusing thoughts and actions allows the thought *'I would go swimming but I have pain'* to change into *'I have pain. I will go swimming.'* The thought *'I have pain'* has become unglued from the valued activity and has lost its power as the reason (barrier) why you did not do what you wanted.

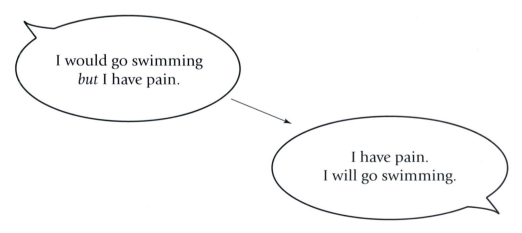

I would go swimming *but* I have pain.

I have pain. I will go swimming.

Speechmark (P) This page may be photocopied for instructional use only © 2014 Keren Fisher and Susan Childs

A TASK FOR YOU

Rate how believable and useful your thought hooks have been this week.

	What thought about pain did your mind produce that hooked you in?	How *believable* was this thought compared with your experience when you obeyed it in the past? *(Measure on a scale of 0–10; 0 = completely believable; 10 = completely unbelievable)*	How *useful* was it in moving you towards your value? *(Measure on a scale of 0–10; 0 = completely useless; 10 = completely useful)*
Day 1			
Day 2			
Day 3			
Day 4			
Day 5			
Day 6			
Day 7			

Speechmark ℗ This page may be photocopied for instructional use only © 2014 Keren Fisher and Susan Childs

TASK

DEFUSION TECHNIQUE: LABELLING THOUGHTS

Thoughts are events in the mind.

Thoughts pass through our minds like cars on a motorway – here and then gone, while others replace them in an endless stream. If we let them pass along, they can't influence our actions. The problem people face with long-term health concerns is that they often stop the line of traffic and *interrogate* a particularly troublesome and persistent thought.

'What if it's true? What if my pain gets worse? What will happen to me if I don't get better?'

This worry process leads to a downward spiral of emotional and behaviour reactions.

You could treat your mind as if it's producing an interesting film and 'watch' the thoughts as they pass through. You could label them like scenes in the film.

'That scene makes me feel anxious and scared.'

Try thinking the thought, *'I would like to go swimming.'*

What is the reaction in your body to that thought?

Does it make you feel anxious about your pain? If so, rather than letting the thought *dictate* your anxious feelings that stop you going swimming, you could label the thought and say:

'There's the thought that makes me feel anxious and scared.'

This alters the thought from a rule into a label. Labels give us information but they do not make us obey them.

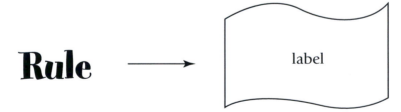

DEFUSION TECHNIQUE: THE SOUND OF PAIN

Words have associations. An example that is often quoted is the word *milk*. Milk is a white, creamy liquid that some people like to drink. Perhaps you had this association when the word was put into your mind. However, it is also just a word.

Try this exercise. Say the word *milk* over and over like this:

milk, milk, milk, milk, milk, milk, milk ... keep going

Speechmark ⑤ Ⓟ This page may be photocopied for instructional use only © 2014 Keren Fisher and Susan Childs

What happens? What did you notice? Sometimes people say that it stops meaning a white, creamy drink and just becomes a strange sound.

In a similar way the word *pain* has associations with suffering, despair, helplessness. The word has become fused to these experiences but it can be just a word that doesn't need to be glued to its evaluations.

Now try this exercise. Say the word pain over and over like this:

pain, pain, pain, pain, pain, pain, pain, pain, pain …

What happens?
What do you notice?
Did the sound of the word stop having its dreaded, familiar meaning?

DEFUSION TECHNIQUE: CARRY THE THOUGHTS WITH YOU WHILE YOU LEAD THE LIFE YOU WANT

Try this exercise.

Write the word PAIN on an index card.

Walk about the room holding the card in front of your eyes.

This is probably not very successful – the word PAIN is stopping you making safe progress across the room. All you can see is PAIN.

Does that sound like your life?

Now put the card in your pocket, or just hold it by your side. Check that you still have it – it hasn't gone away but now you can get on with walking safely to where you want to go.

Your thoughts are like that. If all you can see is the effect of the pain and its associated suffering and loss of a value-led life, you cannot progress in the way you want.

However, you can think of the thoughts as events in the mind and carry them with you while you pursue your valued activities.

Speechmark Ⓟ This page may be photocopied for instructional use only © 2014 Keren Fisher and Susan Childs

DEFUSION TECHNIQUE: THOUGHTS AS PASSENGERS ON THE BUS

You need to imagine that you are driving this bus in the direction of your life value. Perhaps you are going to see about a job. You really want to work and have tried this journey before, but the thought passengers keep doing their best to make you change direction and go home. Usually you obey them and so you have not yet managed to get as far as the job centre. Did your journey look a bit like this?

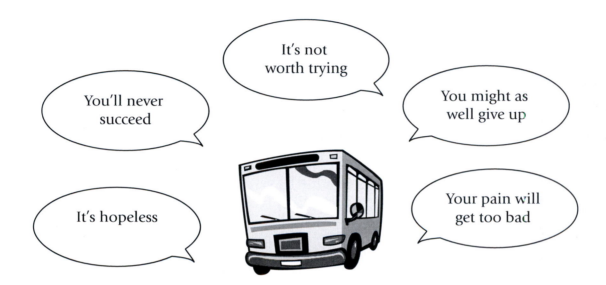

Speechmark Ⓟ This page may be photocopied for instructional use only © 2014 Keren Fisher and Susan Childs

A TASK FOR YOU

Try this exercise with an example from your own life.

You are driving the bus towards your _____ _____ life value.

What did your thought passengers say when you last tried this task? Fill in the speech balloons.

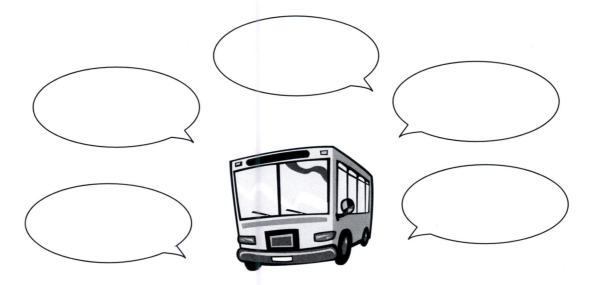

What happened to your journey?

_____

_____

_____

_____

A TASK FOR YOU

This task is about breaking thought habits – getting 'unhooked' from them.

	What was the event that produced the thought?	What thought about pain did your mind produce that hooked you in?	How did you manage to unhook your response from the pain thought? Was this a good or a bad outcome?
Day 1			
Day 2			
Day 3			
Day 4			
Day 5			
Day 6			
Day 7			

Speechmark **P** This page may be photocopied for instructional use only © 2014 Keren Fisher and Susan Childs

Stress and Its Effects on Chronic Pain

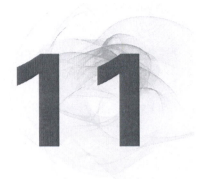

What is the 'stress response'? It is a reaction to an event or situation *you think* you cannot cope with.

> Stress = Demands of situation ÷ the resources you think are available to cope with it.

There are several parts to the stress response: biological, mental, emotional and behavioural.

BIOLOGICAL RESPONSES

The most obvious is probably *biological* – the symptoms you feel straight away, such as increased heart rate, muscle tension and all the other things shown in Figure 1. There are also more hidden effects, such as raised stress hormone levels and a lowered immune system. If you are stressed, you are more likely to catch colds, flu and other bugs.

Where do you feel it?

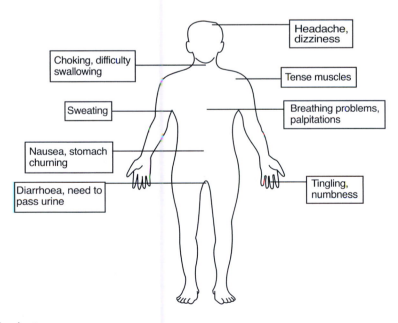

FIGURE 1 Biological stress response

Speechmark (P) This page may be photocopied for instructional use only © 2014 Keren Fisher and Susan Childs

MENTAL RESPONSES

The *mental* response is important in checking the situation for danger. The brain will make a decision and tell the body how to respond. The pituitary gland in the brain directs the adrenal glands in the body to produce adrenalin and cortisol. These prepare the body to speed up and prepare to fight or run away – known as the fight or flight response.

You might also notice that you cannot *think straight or control your thoughts*. Then the reaction can go wrong and the response gets stuck in alarm mode – leading to chronic stress symptoms.

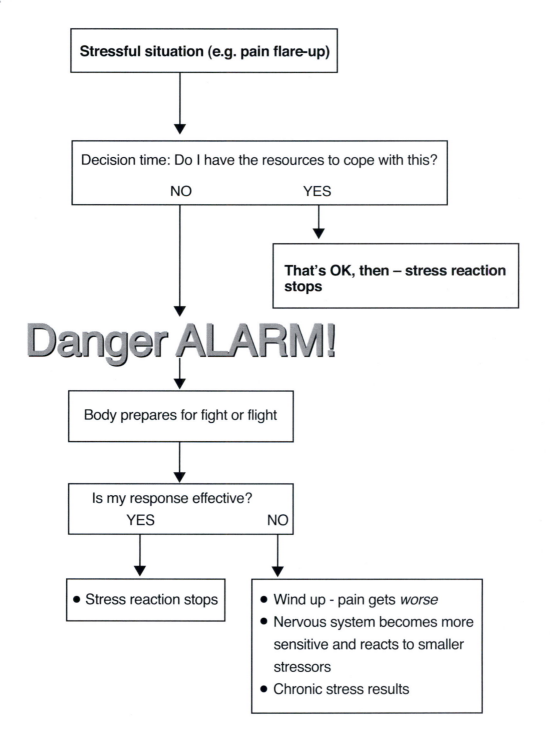

Speechmark ⓢ ⓟ This page may be photocopied for instructional use only © 2014 Keren Fisher and Susan Childs

EMOTIONAL RESPONSES

Emotions are governed by thoughts – by how the brain interprets the situation. You might feel scared, anxious, frustrated, sad, tearful or angry, depending on whether you decided the situation was frightening, depressing or unjust.

BEHAVIOURAL RESPONSES

Emotion will lead to the behavioural response. This might be rushing about, finding lots of unimportant things to do, or feeling too exhausted to do anything at all. It may also result in comfort eating, smoking or drinking alcohol. These are the modern equivalents of 'flight' – using these responses to get away from the experience of stress.

If we think about where these reactions have come from, we might remember our ancient ancestors. According to theories of evolution, it is likely that we are descended from those who had the best stress responses. They were the most successful in dealing with threats from all kinds of challenges in order to survive and pass on their genes.

This was appropriate thousands of years ago when our ancestors had to escape from wild animals. Then, as now, the heart sent more blood to the muscles and diverted it away from digestion, as it was less important. The brain may have had lots of thoughts rushing about which may have helped to form a solution. Sweating allowed the body to cool.

However, the fight or flight response is not really applicable for the type of threats we experience today. Modern stressors do not often need us to respond physically and some of the stress symptoms can mean we experience *more pain*. For example, a sharp intake of breath in response to a large telephone bill might be interpreted as a threat and the brain switches on the stress response, which tenses muscles and increases pain. The fight or flight response, while useful if the threat were actually a tiger, will not help to pay the bill.

BILL	
FINAL DEMAND	£10,000

CAUSES OF STRESS

It is helpful to try to disentangle some of the main sources of stress, rather than think of it as a burden you have to live with all the time, like a big unmanageable black cloud.

Stress might be:
- daily hassles – traffic jams, misbehaving children, delays on buses
- positive life events – parties, weddings, celebrations, holidays
- negative life events – death in the family, divorce, illness, loss of work
- emergencies – accidents, unexpected serious news.

While these things seem to have little in common, in fact they can all be seen as a threat to the person experiencing them. A sense of threat occurs if you believe that the stressor outweighs your coping ability.

Even with 'daily hassles' stress, you might feel the *biological* responses in your body. Your *mental* response might be thoughts such as:

> 'I shall be late if the traffic / children / buses don't hurry up. I might miss my appointment / lose my job. People will be angry with me.'

Your stress response will keep firing and your *emotional* response might be fear, anxiety and frustration. Your *behavioural* response might be to shout at the traffic or the children or the bus driver. Or you might try to rush to make up time and risk falling or making mistakes.

As the stressors become more challenging, you might interpret the threat as *harm*. You believe that damage will happen as a result of the symptoms your body experiences. Your thoughts may become even more distorted. For example, you might think:

> 'My pain is a lot worse now. I must have done something really serious to make it worse than ever.'

Your *emotional* response might be depression and helplessness. Your *behavioural* response might be to reduce physical activity, including work or fitness. This can lead to avoidance of important activities in your value-led life.

Speechmark (P) This page may be photocopied for instructional use only © 2014 Keren Fisher and Susan Childs

STRESS AND AVOIDANCE

The more you avoid something, the more fearful it becomes until stress itself stops you doing it altogether.

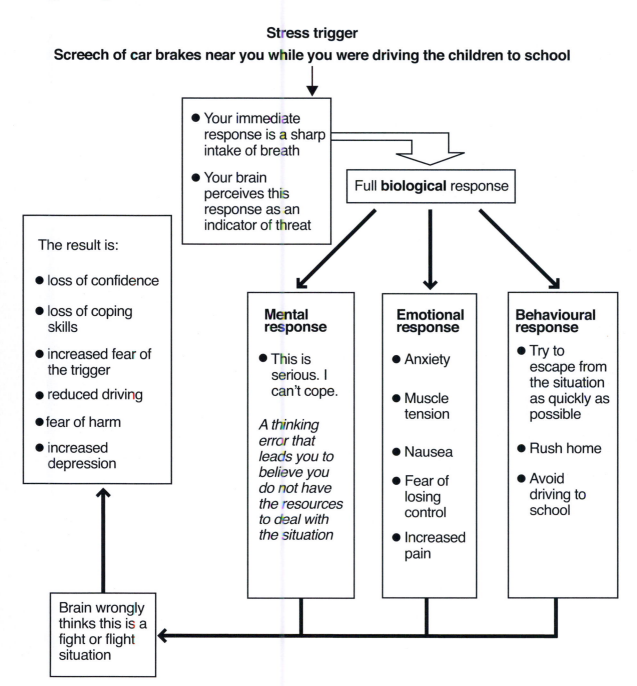

Stress trigger

Screech of car brakes near you while you were driving the children to school

- Your immediate response is a sharp intake of breath
- Your brain perceives this response as an indicator of threat

Full **biological** response

Mental response

- This is serious. I can't cope.

A thinking error that leads you to believe you do not have the resources to deal with the situation

Emotional response

- Anxiety
- Muscle tension
- Nausea
- Fear of losing control
- Increased pain

Behavioural response

- Try to escape from the situation as quickly as possible
- Rush home
- Avoid driving to school

The result is:

- loss of confidence
- loss of coping skills
- increased fear of the trigger
- reduced driving
- fear of harm
- increased depression

Brain wrongly thinks this is a fight or flight situation

TASK

  A TASK FOR YOU

Fill in this table with any stressors you have had this week. Describe what happened in the column you think they fit into. Then record how you felt and what you did.

Day	Daily hassle	Positive life event	Negative life event	Emergency	Your emotional response	Your behavioural response

Speechmark Ⓟ This page may be photocopied for instructional use only © 2014 Keren Fisher and Susan Childs

'FACTOR X'

How does factor X affect your stress?

Some of the things people do when they are stressed are to increase their intake of caffeine, alcohol and other stimulants such as cigarettes or street drugs. These can tip you over into worse stress, as they tend to speed up your heart rate or affect your thinking ability. Even sugary foods can increase stress, as they give you a quick energy boost but leave you depleted afterwards. This fluctuation in blood sugar affects your mood, leaving you tense and less able to deal with the stress that you ate the food to cope with in the first place.

How does factor X affect your pain?

These stimulants or temporary 'stress busters' are the modern version of 'flight' or 'escape' behavioural responses and are largely habits that people might not even be aware they are using. However, as they increase the information flow in the central nervous system, they will have the effect of *opening the pain gates*.

'Factor X'	Effect on body	Effect on pain
Caffeine Alcohol Stimulant drinks Cigarettes Street drugs Sweet foods	Increase in heart rate Increase in muscle tension Increase in neural transmission	Brain receives increased information Brain misinterprets stress symptoms Brain monitors stimuli total and when it exceeds the threshold, the fight or flight response is activated; pain gates open *Pain increases*

Speechmark ⑨ Ⓟ This page may be photocopied for instructional use only © 2014 Keren Fisher and Susan Childs

TASK

  A TASK FOR YOU

Think about your factor X (your 'flight' responses) and tick any in this table that apply to you.

Lots of tea	Lots of coffee	Diet Coke	Stimulant drinks	Cigarettes	Alcohol	Street drugs	Other stimulants	Sweet foods

Can you see where you can reduce your use of these?

_____

_____

_____

_____

What would be the easiest thing to start with?

_____

_____

_____

_____

Speechmark ⓢ Ⓟ This page may be photocopied for instructional use only © 2014 Keren Fisher and Susan Childs

COPING RESOURCES

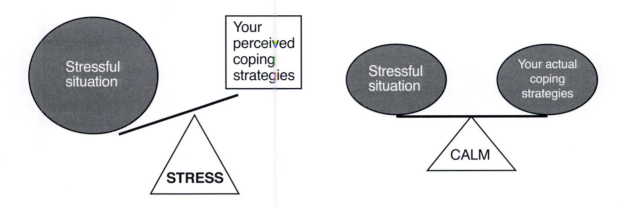

FIGURE 2 Coping with stressful situations

If a situation appears to overwhelm the resources you believe you have to cope with it, then your stress response could act as a *cue* to remind you what strategies you can use to re-evaluate the event. These might be as follows.

1. Looking at your mental interpretation of the event, what is the evidence that it is actually life threatening?
2. Reminding yourself of *mindful breathing*
3. Using *relaxation systems*
4. Using the *four Ps technique*:
    a. Problem solving – look for possible solutions
    b. Prioritising – how important is this today?
    c. Planning – time it for when you are not tired
    d. Pacing – choose a manageable target.

Nancy had to go to a party. Although this was meant to be a positive event, she was dreading meeting people she did not know and having to stand all the evening. As the date got nearer she found herself getting increasingly stressed, until she decided to *practise relaxation* in response to her muscle tension and *challenge her negative mental response* by reminding herself that she could sit down when she needed to and just talk to a few people.

Jim found driving to work stressful. Although it was actually a daily hassle, it seemed to him to be a negative life event and he was aware that his blood pressure was becoming a health hazard. Jim set about solving the problem by *prioritising* leaving for work earlier over an extra fifteen minutes in bed. He *planned* a longer but quieter route and *paced* the journey better by concentrating on *mindful breathing* every time he stopped at traffic lights.

TASK

    A TASK FOR YOU

This exercise is about getting back into balance.

Event	What strategies could you use to switch off the stress response? Mental evaluation? Breathing or relaxation? The four Ps? (Problem solving, Prioritising, Planning, Pacing)

Speechmark P This page may be photocopied for instructional use only © 2014 Keren Fisher and Susan Childs

Relaxation and Chronic Pain

If you are relaxed, then you can't be tense.

Feelings of depression, anger and anxiety can often make your pain worse. One way to reduce the impact of these feelings is by learning to relax various parts of your body. Physical tension – the tightening of muscles – increases physical sensations such as pain. Pain will cause tension and this sets up a vicious circle.

Relaxation can help you stop the pain–tension–anxiety–pain circle.

In fact, there are many ways of relaxing. Some people watch television. Other people read a book. This is fine if it works for you, but most people find *muscle relaxation* is much more effective, as it concentrates directly on the muscle tension component of your pain problem.

Relaxation does several things, as outlined in the following points.

1. Tension and relaxation are opposites. Excessive muscle tension increases the 'work' your muscles are doing. The result is greater fatigue and exhaustion and *more* pain. *Relaxation reduces the amount of pain that is directly caused by tense muscles.*

2. While you are concentrating on relaxing you are *unable to attend much to the experience of pain.* Your brain can only pay attention to so much at one time; therefore, by 'filling it' with relaxation, pain information stays on the edge of your awareness. You will probably still feel your pain but you will find it is not overwhelmingly important. *By occupying your attention with something else, relaxation reduces the amount of pain you experience.*

3. Feelings of depression and anxiety tend to increase muscular tension. This leads to an increase in the pain. *Relaxation reduces feelings of anxiety, frustration and tension and therefore reduces your overall discomfort.*

4. Relaxation exercises help you become aware of and control *specific* muscles that become tense and contribute to your pain. As you practise recognising what your muscles feel like when they are relaxed you will be able to use signs of tenseness as a cue to begin

Speechmark ⬡ Ⓟ This page may be photocopied for instructional use only © 2014 Keren Fisher and Susan Childs relaxation. *Relaxation exercises teach you to recognise tension and respond to it to reduce sensations of pain and fatigue.*

5. Relaxation helps with sleep disturbance that may reduce your capacity to tolerate pain as well as contributing to exhaustion. People often report that it is harder to cope with pain when they are tired, and as the pain gets more difficult to cope with it is harder to sleep. Using relaxation techniques can help reduce the pain and induce sleep, which will further aid your ability to cope with the pain. *Relaxation helps you to sleep and to tolerate your pain better.*

Relaxation is a skill

Learning to relax is the same as learning any other skill – you need practice, just like learning to drive. Practice is best when you're not tensed up – when you feel you least need it. Then, when you know how to relax, you can use it when you need it. This is most important.

Practise when you are not especially tense. Then later you can relax when you feel increased discomfort.

There are different kinds of relaxation instructions, some of which are printed out in this book. Get someone to read the instructions to you and record them onto audiotape or CD or to your personal player. You can also buy lots of different discs and downloads. The best procedure is to find a way to relax your whole body a little at a time. People usually find that it is easier to relax little by little than all at once.

WHERE SHOULD I RELAX?

When you are learning, a quiet place is best to relax. Later on you will be able to relax in other situations. Wear loose clothes and take your shoes off.

You must ensure that you are in the most comfortable position for you – for example, lying on your back on the bed or floor with cushions underneath your neck, knees or back; sitting up in bed; or sitting down on a chair. Everyone is different and what is comfortable to you may not be so for someone else, so think of your individual needs and begin to relax in a comfortable position.

Make sure that you will not be disturbed during the time you are practising. It is difficult to follow the flow and become relaxed if you are interrupted.

Speechmark Ⓟ This page may be photocopied for instructional use only © 2014 Keren Fisher and Susan Childs

HOW OFTEN?

Try to practise at least once a day. Work out the best method for yourself. Then you can relax when you most need it – when you feel increased discomfort and tension in your muscles. Try to recognise the signs of increasing stress and use relaxation as soon as stress starts to build up.

WHAT IF I CAN'T RELAX?

When you begin to relax, your problems may come into your mind. Try to let them drift by, as if you were looking at them from a distance. You can, for example, silently repeat to yourself, 'it doesn't matter'. You may also feel twitches in your muscles. That's perfectly normal. It's the tension being relieved.

Concentration is difficult but it improves with practice. If you are using a recording of the instructions, turn your attention back to it as often as you need to and pick the relaxation up again. The important thing is to learn how to relax and to use the skill whenever you need it.

DIFFERENT WAYS TO RELAX

There are different ways to relax – try them all and choose the one that works best for you.

Diaphragmatic breathing

Diaphragmatic breathing is a very effective way of managing stress as a first response. Use it on its own or with other forms of relaxation.
- When we feel stress, breathing tends to be shallow and we feel dizzy.
- Attend to your breathing and slow it down.
- Make full use of the diaphragm muscle between your chest and your stomach.

Deep muscular relaxation

Deep muscular relaxation helps you to learn the difference between tense and relaxed muscles by tensing first and then relaxing. Many people are not aware of an increase in muscle tension until it actually hurts them.
- Tense the muscles, not so that it hurts but enough so that you can feel the tension. If at any stage you find tensing a certain muscle group increases your pain, then miss this group out. Just concentrate on breathing deeply and slowly in and out and join in the instructions again at the next muscle group.
- Gradually let the tension go and feel the muscles unwind.

Relaxation with imagery

Use this alternative to generate different sensations to counteract some of the characteristics of your pain. Once you have become very experienced at achieving relaxation by a tense and relax method, it is possible to do it more quickly at times when it is inconvenient to sit and concentrate.

- Scan your body for areas of tension and let those areas relax naturally without needing to increase tension first.
- Use breathing to release tension in the shoulders, upper back and chest.
- Think about what the muscles feel like when they are relaxed.

Concentrate on the images that are suggested in the instructions to enhance feelings of relief, refreshment and increased control. Better still, create your own. Some people find that once they have developed useful images, they can 'conjure them up' by turning their attention to these images and this will automatically relax the muscles. It might become a shortcut to the benefits of relaxation.

Differential relaxation: relaxing some parts while using others

Experiment with differential relaxation by walking around the room while keeping your upper body, arms and face relaxed. See how relaxed you can keep all the muscles of your body that are not involved in the activity so that you achieve it with the least effort and discomfort. Make sure you are not gritting your teeth, bracing your knees or clenching your fists.

Build this into your everyday life by trying to make sure that all your actions use no more energy and create no more tension than is needed.

> Practise several times a day, whenever you look at your phone, or take a drink or anything you do at fairly frequent intervals that can act as a reminder.

Speechmark ⑤ ℗ This page may be photocopied for instructional use only © 2014 Keren Fisher and Susan Childs

INSTRUCTIONS FOR RELAXATION TECHNIQUES

Diaphragmatic breathing

- Sit or lie in a comfortable position with your back and neck well supported.
- Put one hand on your abdomen – your stomach area – and the other hand on your chest.
- Take a deep breath in and then let out as much air as possible, letting your shoulders, chest and upper back relax and sink down.
- Breathe in slowly through your nose. Imagine the lowest part of your lungs filled with air. Feel your stomach rise up under your hand. Your stomach should move more than your chest.
- As you breathe out, let your diaphragm relax and feel your stomach sink back under your hand.
- Draw the breath in slowly through your nose and exhale through your mouth, pushing the air out effortlessly.
- Check your chest and stomach movements with your hands.
- Control the rate of breathing by counting seconds, adding the word 'hundred' as you count. This takes roughly one second. Say, 'one hundred, two hundred' etc to yourself.
- Begin a cycle of breathing at the rate of one second in and one second out. Then gradually increase to two seconds in and three seconds out.
- Gradually increase the time taken to breathe in and out – allowing the out breath to take a second longer than the in breath.

It can take a long time to feel confident about controlling your breathing, especially if you have sharp pain or sudden stress. Remember to keep practising so that you are familiar with the technique when you need to use it.

BREATHE

Speechmark Ⓟ This page may be photocopied for instructional use only © 2014 Keren Fisher and Susan Childs

A TASK FOR YOU

Fill in this form to record how helpful breathing practice has been for you.

Day and time	How did you feel before breathing practice?	Pain score before practice (score out of 10)	How did you feel after breathing practice?	Pain score after practice (score out of 10)
Day 1 at:				
Day 2 at:				
Day 3 at:				
Day 4 at:				
Day 5 at:				
Day 6 at:				
Day 7 at:				

Speechmark P This page may be photocopied for instructional use only © 2014 Keren Fisher and Susan Childs

TASK

Deep muscular relaxation

Settle back as comfortably as you can. Let yourself relax as much as possible … Now, as you relax like that, clench your right fist – just clench your fist tighter and tighter, and study the tension as you do so. Keep it clenched and feel the tension in your right fist, hand, forearm … and now relax. Let the fingers of your right hand become loose and observe the contrast in your feelings … Now, let yourself go and try to become more relaxed all over … Now repeat that with your left fist. Clench your left fist while the rest of your body relaxes, clench that fist tighter and feel the tension … and now relax. Enjoy the contrast … Continue relaxing like that for a while … Clench both fists tighter and tighter, both fists tense, forearms tense, study the sensations … and relax, straighten out your fingers and feel that relaxation. Continue relaxing your hands and forearms more and more … Now bend your elbows and tense your biceps, tense them harder and study the tension feelings … Now straighten out your arms, let them relax and feel the difference again. Let the relaxation develop … Each time pay close attention to your feelings when you tense up and when you relax. Now straighten your arms hard, straighten them so that you feel most tension in the triceps muscles along the back of your arms, stretch your arms and feel that tension … and now relax. Get your arms back into a comfortable position. Let the relaxation proceed on its own. The arms should feel comfortably heavy as you allow them to relax … Now let's concentrate on relaxation in the arms without any tension. Get your arms comfortable and let them relax further and further. Continue relaxing your arms even further. Even when your arms seem fully relaxed, try to achieve even deeper levels of relaxation.

Let your muscles go loose and heavy. Just settle back quietly and comfortably. Wrinkle up your forehead now, wrinkle it tighter … and now stop wrinkling your forehead – relax and smooth it out. Picture the entire forehead and scalp becoming smoother as the relaxation increases … Now frown and crease your brows and study the tension … Let go of the tension again … Smooth out the forehead once more … Now, close your eyes tighter and tighter … and feel the tension … and relax your eyes. Keep your eyes closed, gently, comfortably, and notice the relaxation … Now clench your jaw, bite your teeth together, and study the tension throughout the jaw … Relax your jaw now. Let your lips part slightly … Notice the relaxation … Now press your tongue hard against the roof of your mouth. Look for the tension … Now let your tongue return to a comfortable and relaxed position … Now purse your lips, press your lips together tighter and tighter … Relax the lips. Note the contrast between tension and relaxation. Feel the relaxation all over your face, all over your forehead and scalp, eyes, jaw, lips and tongue. The relaxation progresses further and further … Now attend to your neck muscles. Press your head back as far as it can go and feel the tension in the neck, roll it to the right and feel the tension shift, now roll it to the left. Straighten your head and bring it forward, press your chin against your chest … Let your head return to a comfortable position and study the relaxation. Let the relaxation develop. Now shrug your shoulders, right up. Hold the tension … Drop your shoulders and feel the relaxation. Neck and shoulders relaxed … Bring your shoulders up and forward and back. Feel the tension in your shoulders and in your upper back … Drop your shoulders once more and relax.

Relax your entire body as much as you can. Feel the comfortable heaviness that accompanies

Speechmark P This page may be photocopied for instructional use only © 2014 Keren Fisher and Susan Childs

relaxation … Breathe easily and freely in and out. Notice how the relaxation increases as you exhale, as you breathe out just feel the relaxation. Continue relaxing your chest and let the relaxation spread to your back, shoulders, neck and arms. Just let go and enjoy the relaxation. Now pay attention to your abdominal muscles, your stomach area. Tighten your stomach muscles, make your abdomen hard … Notice the tension and relax … Let the muscles loosen and notice the contrast. Notice the general well-being that comes with relaxing your stomach. Now draw your stomach in, pull the muscles right in and feel the tension like this … Now relax again. Let your stomach out … Continue breathing normally and easily and feel the gentle action all over your chest and stomach … Let the tension dissolve as the relaxation grows deeper. Each time you breathe out, notice the rhythmic relaxation in your lungs and your stomach. Notice how your chest and your stomach relax more and more … Now direct your attention to your lower back. Arch up your back, make your lower back quite hollow, and feel the tension along your spine … and settle down comfortably again. Relax the lower back … Try to keep the rest of your body as relaxed as possible … Spread the relaxation to your stomach, chest, shoulders and arms and facial area.

Now tighten your buttocks and thighs. Tighten your thighs by pressing down your knees as hard as you can … Relax and note the difference … Allow the relaxation to proceed on its own … Pull your feet and toes downwards, away from your face, so that your calf muscles become tense. Study that tension … Relax your feet and calves … This time, bend your feet towards your face so that you feel tension along your shins. Bring your toes right up … Relax again. Now let yourself relax further all over. Relax your feet, ankles, calves and shins, knees, thighs, buttocks and hips. Feel the heaviness of your lower body as you relax still further. Feel that relaxation all over. Let it proceed to your upper back, chest, shoulders and arms and right to the tips of your fingers … Make sure that no tension has crept into your throat. Relax your neck and your jaw and all your facial muscles. Keep relaxing your whole body like that for a while. Let yourself relax.

Now you can become twice as relaxed as you are by taking in a really deep breath and slowly exhaling. With your eyes closed so that you become less aware of things around you and so prevent any surface tensions from developing, breathe in deeply and feel yourself becoming heavier. Take in a long, deep breath and let it out very slowly. Feel how heavy and relaxed you have become. Each time you breathe out, relax a little more.

In a state of perfect relaxation you should feel unwilling to move a single muscle in your body. Think about the effort that would be required to answer the phone if it rings. As you think about answering the phone, see if you can notice any tensions that might have crept into your body.

Now decide not to think about the phone ringing but to continue relaxing. Observe the relief and the disappearance of the tension.

Just carry on relaxing like that. When you wish to get up, count backwards from four to one. You should then feel fine and refreshed, wide awake and calm.

RELAX

Speechmark P This page may be photocopied for instructional use only © 2014 Keren Fisher and Susan Childs

A TASK FOR YOU

Fill in this form to record how helpful relaxation practice has been for you.

Day and time	How did you feel before relaxation practice?	Pain score before practice (score out of 10)	How did you feel after relaxation practice?	Pain score after practice (score out of 10)
Day 1 at:				
Day 2 at:				
Day 3 at:				
Day 4 at:				
Day 5 at:				
Day 6 at:				
Day 7 at:				

Speechmark ⓟ This page may be photocopied for instructional use only © 2014 Keren Fisher and Susan Childs

Relaxation with imagery: warm version

Have your legs outstretched and uncrossed with your arms by your sides. Close your eyes and let yourself become as comfortable as you can. Relax as deeply as you can. Let all the tensions ease away from your body, comfortable and relaxed. No tension anywhere in your body.

Think of your hands and arms. Try to feel whether there is any tension present and if there is, then try to relax that little bit more.

And think about your shoulders. If there is any tension in your shoulders then try to note where it is and relax that tension.

Now attend to the muscles in your neck. Make sure that they are relaxed. Make sure that your head is in a comfortable position, well supported, so that you can let go any tension in your neck.

Think about the muscles of your face, your forehead. If there is any tension in your forehead then try to let it relax and ease away.

And the muscles around your eyes, make sure that your eyelids are just lightly closed with no pressure, no effort.

Now think about the muscles around your mouth and jaw, make sure that your teeth are slightly parted so that there is no tension or pressure between your lips, your lips just lightly together. And notice your tongue and throat. Make sure that they are relaxed.

Make sure that the muscles of your chest are relaxed. Keep your breathing nice and even but not too deep. Every time you breathe out imagine saying the word 'relax' under your breath. Each time you say the word 'relax' try to feel the muscles of your chest relax that little bit more. Relax that little bit more.

And think about the muscles of your stomach. If you feel any tension in the muscles of your stomach then try to let them relax and unwind.

Now attend to the muscles of your legs, if there is any tension in your legs then try to feel where the tension is and relax it. No tension in your legs, just deeper and deeper relaxation.

Try to feel your whole body become more and more deeply relaxed. Enjoy the feeling of letting go. Feel the pleasant sensation of heaviness as you let the muscles relax and unwind.

Now imagine taking four steps, with each step becoming more and more heavy and relaxed. Imagine the first step, feeling heavy and relaxed, and the second step, very heavy and relaxed, and the third step, even more heavy and relaxed and the fourth step, very heavy and comfortable and relaxed. Let the feelings of heaviness and relaxation increase and focus on the thought, 'My body feels heavy and relaxed'.

Now imagine a pleasant scene in which you would feel as completely relaxed as you are now. Perhaps a warm, sunny summer's day or listening to a favourite piece of music. Imagine that scene clearly now and try to feel the feeling of relaxation that you associate with that scene. Feel yourself relaxing more and more deeply, just letting go more and more.

Speechmark P This page may be photocopied for instructional use only © 2014 Keren Fisher and Susan Childs

Imagine lying in the sun. Concentrate on the feelings of heat and notice how warm your skin feels as it absorbs the heat of the sun. The warmer your skin feels, the more comfortable and relaxed you become. Focus on the thought, 'My skin feels warm' and let the process continue as far as you want … Think about removing all sensations of tension and discomfort and letting warmth and relaxation take their place. Focus on the thought, 'My body feels warm and comfortable'.

Now imagine being in a warm bath or shower. Feel the sensations of warmth on your skin. Think about the warmth of the water taking away feelings of tension and discomfort … Focus on the thought, 'My skin feels warm' and let the process continue as far as you want … Let the feelings of warmth increase and the warmer your skin feels, the more relaxed and comfortable you become. Focus on the thought, 'My body feels warm and comfortable'.

From time to time your mind will wander. This is completely normal. Don't fight it. Just gently return to your mental image and try to feel your whole body relax that little bit more. Don't feel you have to work too hard at it. If your mind wanders, just gently guide it back to your mental image. Try to feel your body relax as you do so.

Imagine your areas of discomfort becoming smaller and smaller as your body feels warm and more relaxed. Let the process continue as far as you want … The more comfortable and relaxed you become, the smaller your remaining areas of discomfort can grow … Let the feelings of warmth and relaxation take the place of feelings of discomfort and tension. Focus on the thought, 'My body feels warm, comfortable and relaxed'.

Concentrate on the words 'relax' and 'warm'. Use these words whenever you feel pain and discomfort. Use the word 'relax' to become relaxed and comfortable. Use the word 'warm', to increase feelings of warmth and comfort taking the place of feelings of discomfort.

When you want to get up, think about taking your four steps back again, and with each step becoming more alert and awake … Think about the fourth step and the third step, becoming more alert and awake now, and the second step, quite alert and awake, and the first step, alert, awake and comfortable.

WARM

TASK

    A TASK FOR YOU

Fill in this form to record how helpful imagery practice has been for you.

Day and time	How did you feel before imagery practice?	Pain score before practice (score out of 10)	How did you feel after imagery practice?	Pain score after practice (score out of 10)
Day 1 at:				
Day 2 at:				
Day 3 at:				
Day 4 at:				
Day 5 at:				
Day 6 at:				
Day 7 at:				

Speechmark P This page may be photocopied for instructional use only © 2014 Keren Fisher and Susan Childs

Relaxation with imagery: cool version

Have your legs outstretched and uncrossed with your arms by your sides. Close your eyes and let yourself become as comfortable as you can. Relax as deeply as you can. Let all the tensions ease away from your body, comfortable and relaxed. No tension anywhere in your body.

Think of your hands and arms. Try to feel whether there is any tension present and if there is, then try to relax that little bit more.

And think about your shoulders. If there is any tension in your shoulders then try to note where it is and relax that tension.

Now attend to the muscles in your neck. Make sure that they are relaxed. Make sure that your head is in a comfortable position, well supported, so that you can let go any tension in your neck.

Think about the muscles of your face, your forehead. If there is any tension in your forehead then try to let it relax and ease away.

And the muscles around your eyes, make sure that your eyelids are just lightly closed with no pressure, no effort.

Now think about the muscles around your mouth and jaw, make sure that your teeth are slightly parted so that there is no tension or pressure between your lips, your lips just lightly together. And your tongue and throat, make sure that they are relaxed.

Make sure that the muscles of your chest are relaxed. Keep your breathing nice and even but not too deep. Every time you breathe out imagine saying the word 'relax' under your breath. Each time you say the word 'relax' try to feel the muscles of your chest relax that little bit more. Relax that little bit more.

And think about the muscles of your stomach. If you feel any tension in the muscles of your stomach then try to let them relax and unwind.

Now attend to the muscles of your legs, if there is any tension in your legs then try to feel where the tension is and relax it. No tension in your legs, just deeper and deeper relaxation.

Try to feel your whole body become more and more deeply relaxed. Enjoy the feeling of letting go. Feel the pleasant sensation of heaviness as you let the muscles relax and unwind.

Now imagine taking four steps, with each step becoming more and more heavy and relaxed. Imagine the first step, feeling heavy and relaxed, and the second step, very heavy and relaxed, and the third step, even more heavy and relaxed and the fourth step, very heavy and comfortable and relaxed. Let the feelings of heaviness and relaxation increase and focus on the thought, 'My body feels heavy and relaxed'.

Now imagine a pleasant scene in which you would feel as completely relaxed as you are now. Perhaps you're walking through a forest or listening to a favourite piece of music. Imagine that scene clearly now and try to feel the feeling of relaxation that you associate with that scene. Feel yourself relaxing more and more deeply, just letting go more and more.

Now imagine what it feels like to be in a cool shower on a hot day. Concentrate on the feelings of coolness, of being refreshed and cool and comfortable. Imagine yourself in the shower and turning the temperature of the water down until it feels cool, comfortable and refreshing. The cooler your skin feels, the more comfortable and relaxed you become. Focus on the thought, 'My skin feels cool' and let the process continue as far as you want … Think about removing all sensations of tension and discomfort and letting coolness and relaxation take their place. Focus on the thought, 'My body feels cool and comfortable'.

Now think about what it's like to be in a cool breeze on a hot day. Think about the sensations of the breeze on your skin … Imagine the cool breeze taking the place of burning discomfort … Focus on the thought, 'My skin feels cool' and let the process continue as far as you want … Just let the cool breeze refresh you and the more cool and refreshed you feel, the more relaxed and comfortable you become. Focus on the thought, 'My body feels cool and comfortable'.

From time to time your mind will wander. This is completely normal. Don't fight it. Just gently return to your mental image and try to feel your whole body relax that little bit more. Don't feel you have to work too hard at it. If your mind wanders, just gently guide it back to your mental image. Try to feel your body relax as you do so.

Imagine your areas of discomfort becoming smaller and smaller as your body feels cool and more relaxed. Let the process continue as far as you want … The more comfortable and relaxed you become, the smaller your remaining areas of discomfort can grow … Let the feelings of coolness and relaxation take the place of feelings of discomfort and tension. Focus on the thought, 'My body feels cool, comfortable and relaxed'.

Concentrate on the words 'relax' and 'cool'. Use these words whenever you feel pain and discomfort. Use the word 'relax' to become relaxed and comfortable. Use the word 'cool', to increase feelings of coolness and refreshment taking the place of feelings of burning and discomfort.

When you want to get up, think about taking your four steps back again, and with each step becoming more alert and awake … Think about the fourth step and the third step, becoming more alert and awake now, and the second step, quite alert and awake, and the first step, alert, awake and comfortable.

COOL

Speechmark P This page may be photocopied for instructional use only © 2014 Keren Fisher and Susan Childs

A TASK FOR YOU

Fill in this form to record how helpful imagery practice has been for you.

Day and time	How did you feel before imagery practice?	Pain score before practice (score out of 10)	How did you feel after imagery practice?	Pain score after practice (score out of 10)
Day 1 at:				
Day 2 at:				
Day 3 at:				
Day 4 at:				
Day 5 at:				
Day 6 at:				
Day 7 at:				

Speechmark Ⓟ This page may be photocopied for instructional use only © 2014 Keren Fisher and Susan Childs

Differential relaxation

Relax as deeply as you can. Let all the tensions ease away from your body, comfortable and relaxed. No tension anywhere in your body.

Now think about the muscles in your fingers. Move your fingers while keeping the rest of your body completely relaxed. Concentrate on the sensations of moving your fingers while keeping the rest of your body relaxed and comfortable. And now relax your hands again.

Now bend your arms at the elbows and raise your hands in the air. Raise your hands and make waving movements. Move your hands but keep the rest of your body relaxed. Concentrate on how it feels to move one part of your body while keeping the rest completely relaxed.

Now relax your arms again. No tension in your hands or arms. Just let the whole of your body relax completely.

And now, while keeping the rest of your body completely relaxed, open your eyes and look around you. Move your eyes around while keeping the rest of your body completely relaxed. Just move your eyes and keep everything else still. Notice how it feels to move your eyes while keeping the rest of your body completely relaxed. Now move your head slightly from side to side and carry on looking around you, keeping the movements slow, steady and relaxed.

Now stop moving your head. Let your head and neck relax again completely.

Now slowly, sit upright keeping your shoulders relaxed, your neck and your stomach relaxed. Now stretch your muscles, get up slowly and stand in a relaxed position. Make sure that you can stand with the whole of your body relaxed. The only work you need is in the muscles of your legs, abdomen and back. Make sure you're not bracing your knees, hunching your shoulders or gritting your teeth.

Now walk slowly around the room. Take a few steps walking slowly and comfortably. Notice how you can walk and yet keep your body relaxed, using only the muscles necessary for the movements you are making. Keep your movements slow so that they are relaxed and easy. No tension in your arms, shoulders, neck or face. No tension in your chest or stomach. Notice how you can carry out this action and yet stay relaxed and comfortable.

Now sit down again. Settle back comfortably and relaxed. Let your whole body relax completely once again.

When you are ready, get up slowly, remembering to keep as relaxed as possible.

RELAX

Speechmark   Ⓟ This page may be photocopied for instructional use only © 2014 Keren Fisher and Susan Childs

A TASK FOR YOU

Fill in this form to record how helpful relaxation practice has been for you.

Day and time	How did you feel before relaxation practice?	Pain score before practice (score out of 10)	How did you feel after relaxation practice?	Pain score after practice (score out of 10)
Day 1 at:				
Day 2 at:				
Day 3 at:				
Day 4 at:				
Day 5 at:				
Day 6 at:				
Day 7 at:				

Speechmark P This page may be photocopied for instructional use only © 2014 Keren Fisher and Susan Childs

Sleep and Chronic Pain

13

It is important to remember that there is no such thing as 'a proper amount of sleep'. The body decides how much it needs depending on how much it has been active during the day and how much sleep you have had in recent nights.

People tend to sleep more than they think they do, but it is the *quality* of sleep that might give the impression of a bad night.

'Normal' sleep cycles occur about every 60–100 minutes throughout the night and follow a pattern of stages (*see* Figure 1).

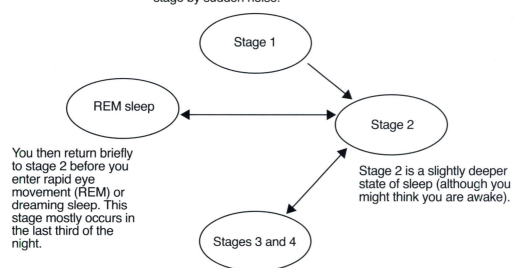

Stage 1 is light sleep: a drowsy and relaxed state between sleeping and waking when the heart rate and blood pressure drop and the muscles relax. You can be easily awakened in this stage by sudden noise.

You then return briefly to stage 2 before you enter rapid eye movement (REM) or dreaming sleep. This stage mostly occurs in the last third of the night.

Stage 2 is a slightly deeper state of sleep (although you might think you are awake).

Stages 3 and 4 are deep sleep, when it is very difficult to be woken and if you are disturbed you'll be confused and disorientated because blood has been diverted from the brain to your muscles. This stage mostly occurs in the first third of the night.

FIGURE 1 Stages of sleep

Speechmark Ⓟ This page may be photocopied for instructional use only © 2014 Keren Fisher and Susan Childs

SLEEP CYCLES CHANGE THROUGHOUT THE NIGHT

As people enter stage 1 sleep they are sometimes aware of the changes in their brain wave pattern and relaxation in their muscles. They can experience a jolt like falling from a height. *This is normal and harmless.*

During the night the cycles repeat, beginning again at stage 2 after a REM sleep episode. Sometimes people wake briefly, remembering their dreams but also being aware that they cannot move, as the muscles are paralysed in REM sleep.

Throughout the night the time you spend in each stage changes. There is more deep sleep early in the night and more REM and light sleep later, which may explain why you are more aware of light sleep in the morning and believe you have not slept well.

You may also wake for an hour or two about four hours after you first fell asleep. While this might be annoying, it is very common, especially in older people, and in people who believe they only need four hours' sleep. These people do not return for a 'second sleep' later in the night.

In the days of our ancestors, before the origin of streetlights and night-time activities, it was the normal pattern for people to go to sleep soon after dark and to then be awake for an hour or two about four hours later, before they returned to sleep for a second sleep phase. People used to get up for a while, and physicians encouraged them to have sex at this time as it was said to be more satisfying than after a day's activity. If this is your pattern, it is considered *completely natural*. You could follow the old advice!

However, it is important not to switch on your television, computer or mobile phone at this time, as exposure to too much artificial light will inhibit the production of the hormone melatonin, which makes you feel sleepy. Artificial light of this kind will stimulate the brain to wake up and will make returning to sleep for the second period more difficult. You could also avoid caffeine and alcoholic drinks for the same reason. Alcohol initially acts as a stimulant before it depresses critical brain areas involved in making good plans.

If you normally take medication if you wake at about 0300, you must be sure that this is part of your recommended 24-hour allowance and *not an extra dose*.

PROBLEMS WITH SLEEP AND PAIN

People who have pain often develop sleep problems because of muscle tension, low mood and lack of physical activity during the day. This can then form a vicious circle in which the effects of poor sleep make the whole situation more distressing. Figure 2 shows what the problem can tend to look like.

Speechmark ⓟ This page may be photocopied for instructional use only © 2014 Keren Fisher and Susan Childs

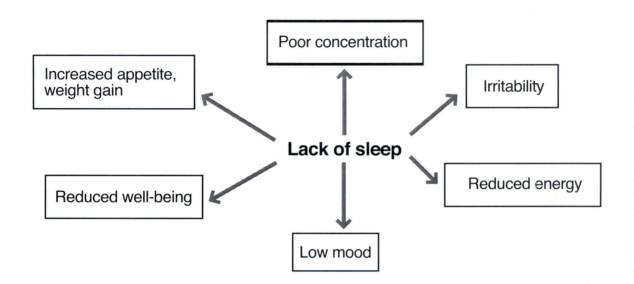

FIGURE 2 Lack of sleep

And the sum total equals:

pain feels worse and is harder to live with.

So, you need a plan to minimise an actual lack of sleep, while remembering that it is not essential to be asleep for a continuous seven or eight hours.

- **Make sure your room and bed are comfortable**. Use a memory foam mattress topper if necessary.
- **Establish a regular routine**. Go to bed and, more important, *get up* at the same time every day regardless of how much sleep you have had. Bodies like habits and if you get up late, you'll develop a habit of moving the onset of your sleep cycle to early morning instead of at night.
- **Your bed should only be associated with sleep and sex**. Apart from reducing the sleepy effects of melatonin, watching television or working in bed will break the association between going to bed and falling asleep. Your bed should act as a powerful cue for sleep, like a bus is a cue for travelling somewhere.
- **Don't *try* to sleep**. If you are not asleep within about 20 minutes, get up, go into another room and read in a soft light until you feel ready to sleep. This will save you worrying about not being asleep. Go to bed later if necessary, but still get up at a set time. This will gradually adjust your sleep cycle.
- **Relaxation techniques**. Use relation techniques to help you prepare for sleep. Attention to your breathing and creating feelings of heaviness in your muscles will help you to feel sleepy. It will also help with feelings of anxiety and depression, although if you're very stressed you may need to work on solving the problem first.

Speechmark P This page may be photocopied for instructional use only © 2014 Keren Fisher and Susan Childs

A TASK FOR YOU

Fill in this sleep diary every morning by estimating the time you are awake and asleep. This will help you to identify where you need to make changes.

Time	Day 1	Day 2	Day 3	Day 4	Day 5	Day 6	Day 7
Went to bed							
Fell asleep							
Woke up: ● first ● second ● third							
Activities while awake *For example:* ● *Got up* ● *Watched television* ● *Read* ● *Practised relaxation*							
Went back to sleep: ● second ● third ● fourth							
Woke finally							
Got up							

Can you see where you can make changes? What would be easiest to start with?

_____

_____

_____

_____

Speechmark ⑤ Ⓟ This page may be photocopied for instructional use only © 2014 Keren Fisher and Susan Childs

Relationships, Communication and Intimacy in Chronic Pain

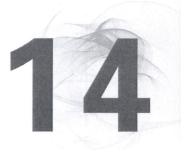

You do not experience your pain in a vacuum. There are other people in your life who are affected too. They may even share whatever emotional reactions you have towards your situation.

If you feel *helpless* about coping, people who care about you will not know what to do either. They will try to make it better for you, but their efforts will not necessarily address what you need.

If you feel *guilty* about expecting your family and friends to put up with you, they can feel equally guilty about being unable to make you feel better.

If you feel *anxious* about whether your partner will leave you if you do not improve, your partner might feel equally anxious about how the relationship can survive if you stay together.

Some people may disappear altogether just to get out of the spiral of failure and depression. At the point when you think you most need them, the very people you require seem to abandon you.

Looking at things from their point of view can get friends and family to help you cope, which involves being very specific about what you are asking them to do.

Mind reading doesn't work, in spite of what television programmes tell us!

If they say, *'Let me know if there's anything I can do'*, you could assume they don't really mean it or they would be doing something useful already, *or* you could say, *'It would be great if you could help me bring the shopping in from the car.'*

If they say, *'I wish there was something I could say to make you feel better'*, you could sigh deeply, *or* you could say, *'Let's talk about yesterday's soap episode / concert / film'* (or whatever interest you have in common).

If your partner says, *'I feel anxious about how we can stay together unless we can work something out'*, you could say, *'Perhaps you should leave if that's what you want'*, *or*

 Speechmark ⓟ This page may be photocopied for instructional use only © 2014 Keren Fisher and Susan Childs

you could say, *'Let's go for a nice meal and discuss how we can still do the things we enjoy, even if more slowly.'*

All these responses depend on your being upfront and assertive about what you want the others to do in order for you all to cope better.

Assertiveness allows you to express your *feelings, needs, rights and opinions* in ways that empower you and strengthen your belief that you have a valuable contribution to make regardless of other people's views.

> If you're interested to see how assertive you are, visit www.queendom.com and scroll down to 'Attitude & Lifestyle tests …'.

ASSERTIVENESS IN MORE DETAIL: THE EFFECT OF COMMUNICATION STYLE ON YOUR PAIN.

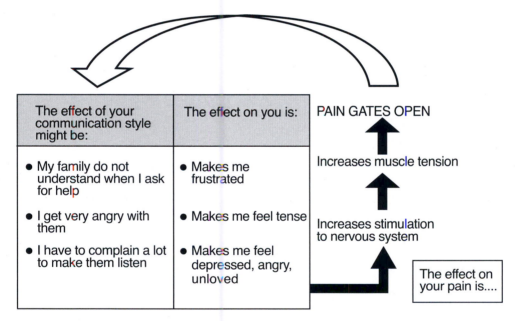

The effect of your communication style might be:	The effect on you is:
• My family do not understand when I ask for help	• Makes me frustrated
• I get very angry with them	• Makes me feel tense
• I have to complain a lot to make them listen	• Makes me feel depressed, angry, unloved

PAIN GATES OPEN

Increases muscle tension

Increases stimulation to nervous system

The effect on your pain is....

This indicates that the way some people communicate to others about their pain may end up making the situation a whole lot worse.

Communication styles fall into three broad categories.

1. *Passive* – poor eye contact, apologetic, quiet, defensive body posture, uses 'I'm sorry …' statements, puts others' needs ahead of own
2. *Assertive* – comfortable eye contact, good listening, upright confident body posture, uses 'I think … I would like …' statements, acknowledges the balance between own and others' needs, states own needs clearly
3. *Aggressive* – excessive eye contact, invades other people's space, loud, confrontational body posture, uses 'You make me …' statements, puts own needs ahead of the needs of others.

Tone of voice is a good indicator of the prominent style, but this varies with the circumstances. A 'bad pain day' may change you from your usual, nicely assertive style into one or both of the others – *passive* if you tend to go quiet with pain, or *aggressive* if you tend to feel frustrated and angry.

> Your pain might trip you into using a style that's not normally yours.

EVENTS THAT TRIP YOU OUT OF YOUR ASSERTIVE STYLE

If we imagine that there is a continuum from a passive to an aggressive style and that assertiveness falls somewhere in the middle, you might rate yourself as a fairly assertive but quite peaceable person like the 'x' on the line.

Passive Assertive   Aggressive

⌐ _ _ _ _ _ _ x _ _ ⌐ _ _ _ _ _ _ _ _ _ _ ⌐

Now let us assume that one day you wake up in terrible pain and struggle all morning (despite painkillers) to get on top of it. At lunchtime family members ask you to help them decorate the living room. What response will you make?

A. You agree to help even though secretly you know it will be a bad idea (you trip into an initially passive style).

B. You refuse to help and tell your family that they should know that your pain does not allow you do this kind of activity (you trip into an aggressive style).

C. You explain that although you can see they need your help, today is a bad pain day so you can only offer a short spell at a physically easy task (staying with an assertive style).

While C is probably the best response, it may not spring to mind automatically. Either of the other responses will have an effect a bit like that shown in Figure 1.

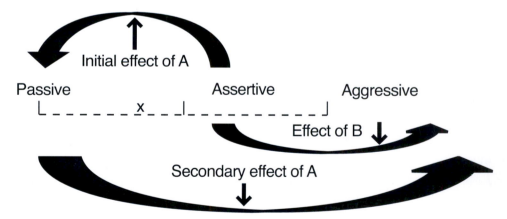

FIGURE 1 Responses on the passive–aggressive continuum

It seems that even if you try to do what they want, you still end up feeling angry and aggressive. Why is that?

Speechmark   P This page may be photocopied for instructional use only © 2014 Keren Fisher and Susan Childs

A passive style fails to acknowledge your own needs and you end up feeling exploited and undervalued. Eventually this will flip you into aggressiveness as a self-protection strategy.

EFFECT OF AGGRESSIVE STYLE ON PAIN EXPERIENCE

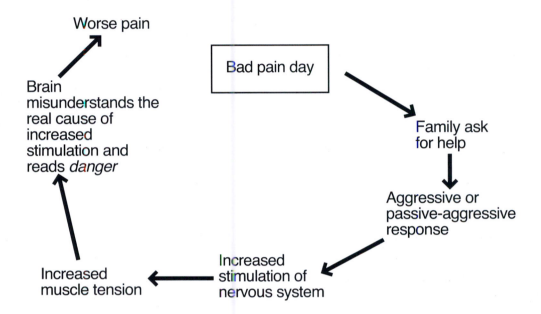

FIGURE 2 Pain experience with aggressive style

As the brain has increased its pain messages to alert you to take action against possible danger, the whole event outlined in Figure 2 seems to have spiralled out of control.

What would help to reduce the impact of this communication style on the pain level?

> Assertiveness recognises the balance between your own needs and those of others.

Use the three-point plan

1. Acknowledge the needs of the others (help with decorating)
2. Acknowledge your need (must take it slowly today)
3. Negotiate a solution (you suggest offering a short spell at a physically easy task)

This approach has the effect of *reducing* the potential threat to everyone concerned.

- Your family are happy that you want to make an effort for them.
- You are confident about what you can achieve without increasing your pain still further.
- The decorating makes progress.

 P This page may be photocopied for instructional use only © 2014 Keren Fisher and Susan Childs

A CLOSER LOOK AT ASSERTIVENESS SKILLS

Saying 'no' can be a challenge, but it is important if we want to avoid doing things we don't want to do. We might think it seems mean or selfish but in fact, it is better to be straight-forward (although not rude) and tell the other person if we find their request too difficult. Communicating assertively can help.

Start with some foundations
- Identify the emotions you noticed in the situation
- Identify what you agreed with and did not agree with about the situation
- Plan with what or where you would be happy to compromise
- Plan the best words to say in the situation
- Plan the best time to say them

Add some listening skills
- Focus on the other person or people
- Make good eye contact
- Stand with open body language and posture
- Use verbal prompts: *'hmm, oh dear, yes, I see …'*
- Use open-ended questions: *'What? When? Where? How?'*
- Use reflection phrases: *'Oh, I see, you're saying …'*

Avoid
- Responding in anger
- Being manipulative: *'you're so nice generally but …'*
- Giving unrealistic assurance that everything will be all right
- Changing the subject

Try to agree where you can
- Agree with some aspects if you believe them: *'Yes, that's true. Sometimes I …'*
- Try to get specific examples: *'Can you give me an example of when I …'*

Negotiate a realistic compromise
- Be clear about your desired outcome
- Investigate the other person's goal fully
- Bear in mind any time limits
- Be as flexible as you can

  This page may be photocopied for instructional use only © 2014 Keren Fisher and Susan Childs

OTHER APPROACHES TO REDUCING THE IMPACT OF UNHELPFUL COMMUNICATION ON PAIN

Strategy	Why?
Diaphragmatic breathing	Helps control muscle tension in shoulders, chest and neck Helps control tone of voice
Regular relaxation practice	Keeps general level of muscle tension down; this reduces the overall level of stimulation
Practise *using* 'I think ...', 'I like ...' statements	Helps to convey responsibility for your needs
Practise *avoiding* 'I'm sorry ...' statements	These convey passiveness and helplessness and make it more likely that your needs will not be met
Practise *avoiding* 'You make me ...' statements	These convey aggression and lack of respect for others' needs; anger and frustration will escalate
Practise open, upright, confident body posture, not too distant, nor too confrontational	Helps to get your point across without being apologetic or too insistent
Explain your 'pain tone' (extra quiet or extra irritable) to others	The tone related to your pain might not be recognised by others and may be misinterpreted
Ask for time to consider requests and demands from others	Allows for planning and better communication style
Practise finding an assertive response	Helps you bring the most effective response to mind more easily
Cognitive behavioural therapy thought challenging	Helps you to step back from the situation – this helps you to question your automatic response
Mindfulness	Allows you to unhook from your emotional response; lets you observe your reaction and allows you to consider your options

WE ALSO NEED TO UNDERSTAND THE EFFECT OF THESE DIFFERENT COMMUNICATION STYLES ON THE LISTENER

Consider the examples outlined in this table.

Situation	Passive (fail to acknowledge your needs)	Aggressive (fail to acknowledge others' needs)	Assertive [(1) acknowledge others' needs; (2) acknowledge your needs; (3) negotiate a solution]
You have agreed to go on a weekend trip but now you are unsure you will manage.	It's a bad time for me, but I'll come anyway. I don't want to let the others down.	I'm not coming. You shouldn't have asked me. If you want me to come you should have arranged a more convenient trip.	Yes, it's more fun if we're all together (1), but I'm not sure I'll be able to do the whole weekend (2). Would it be best if I make my own travel arrangements so as not to put you all out if I have to leave early? (3)
It is 1600 on Friday and your boss asks you to do more work. You feel stressed enough already.	OK. I'll stay and get it finished. I'll have the weekend to recover.	There's no way I can do that. You've made me feel too stressed this week already. At this rate you'll give me no alternative but to resign.	Yes, I can see this is urgent (1), but I won't be able to finish it all today (2). Could you reduce it a bit or could you get someone else to help me? (3)

How would your friends respond to your *passive* reply to the weekend trip, or your boss to the extra work? Most likely they would just accept that you were able to do what they wanted. They would fail to notice that your pain problem needed consideration. You might feel increasingly unsupported and eventually quite *angry* or *depressed*.

Alternatively, what might be the reaction to your *aggressive* responses? Your friends are unlikely to want to invite you again and may well drift away from you altogether, leaving you miserable and isolated. Your boss might well consider getting rid of you, as you seem so inflexible and unhelpful. Losing your job might result in depression, anger and anxiety.

These emotional reactions are all extra stimulation to the nervous system and will tend to be interpreted in the brain as *more pain*.

Assertively stating your own needs while understanding theirs will reduce the emotional temperature and help to prevent an increase in pain.

Speechmark Ⓟ This page may be photocopied for instructional use only © 2014 Keren Fisher and Susan Childs

A TASK FOR YOU

Try this exercise using an example from your own life.

Situation:

What outcome did you want?	What would be the *passive* response?	What would be the *aggressive* response?	What would be the *assertive* response?

How have you responded to this situation in the past?

Did you give a passive response? (Yes or no)
If *yes*, what was the outcome?

_____

_____

_____

_____

Did you give an aggressive response? (Yes or no)
If *yes*, what was the outcome?

_____

_____

_____

Did you give an assertive response? (Yes or no)
If *yes*, what was the outcome?

_____

_____

_____

This page may be photocopied for instructional use only © 2014 Keren Fisher and Susan Childs

COMMUNICATING IN OTHER TYPES OF RELATIONSHIPS

You might recognise people like those in the table here and 'feel' their implied message. You could try responding in the assertive ways like those suggested here and *hope you can get on their wavelength*.

Roles taken by 'friends':	What they say:	Message:	You feel:	You could say:
Criticiser	It's your own fault if the pain's worse. You shouldn't have done so much yesterday.	You are to blame	Guilty	Yes. It would be better if we agreed the rules for pacing and stuck to them.
Fixer	You should try my grandmother's technique. Or there's always a better painkiller. You only have to ask.	You are not trying hard enough	Incompetent	Yes, thanks for the suggestion. I've tried all the pills there are and have the best ones at the moment.
Competitor	At least you can walk. My pain's so bad I can hardly move.	You make too much fuss	Undermined	Yes, that's true. I'm sorry it's so bad for you. Let's just sit and rest for a bit.
Sympathiser	You're so brave. It must be dreadful for you. Never mind, it'll soon be better.	You just need reassurance	Infantilised	Yes, it was bad at first. I'm getting used to coping now.
Entertainer	Cheer up. I know a few good jokes to make you forget about it.	You are too depressing to be around	Misunderstood	Yes, thank you. I could do with a bit of fun occasionally.

But if none of this helps to move these friendships along and they still make you feel dragged down rather than motivated, it may be best to reduce your contact with these friends. If you have limited energy, you need to focus your effort where it will be most rewarded. Some pain patients say such friendships should be 'culled'.

Speechmark Ⓢ Ⓟ This page may be photocopied for instructional use only © 2014 Keren Fisher and Susan Childs

COMMUNICATION AND INTIMACY IN CHRONIC PAIN

Many couples live full and contented lives without sex in their relationship. While it is important for many, sex may not be the primary concern for you. Still, some type of physical intimacy is often comforting and it is reassuring that you can make changes to work around your pain if you can put in the time and commitment.

Sometimes sexual activity, even just hugging and kissing, can increase pain. This may then lead to difficulties in the relationship in general, and if there were sexual problems before the onset of your pain problem, the pain itself may have made them worse. These will soon start to affect you, your partner and your family.

One common way of dealing with such problems is to avoid sex.

What would be the negative consequences of avoidance?
- Over time, avoidance of sex can lead to avoidance of all physical closeness.
- Avoidance can lead to tension and anxiety.
- Avoidance can lead to relationship difficulties – perceived or actual rejection.
- Avoiding sexual activity can result in difficulties when trying to start a new relationship.

Before you start thinking about making changes, it is worth considering where the problem really lies.

Is your chronic pain the root of this sexual problem or is there something else?

Are you worrying excessively about your partner's needs in other areas of the relationship?

The most important step is *communication*.

It is hard to solve anything without talking it over. This is a shared problem. If you need to explore relationship problems in general, it may be easier if you approach a counselling service.

Even if you are single, counselling can help you, and it is always useful to learn as much as possible about how to achieve the best, most fulfilling relationship you can.

Common thoughts about intimacy reported by pain patients and their partners

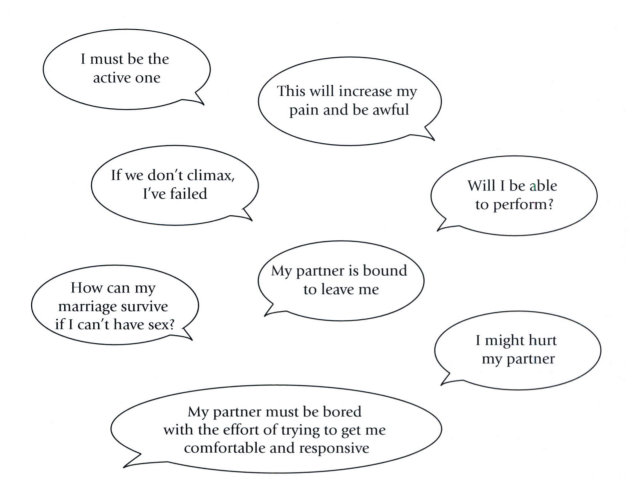

Do you recognise any of these thoughts? What is the evidence they are true?

Speechmark ⓟ This page may be photocopied for instructional use only © 2014 Keren Fisher and Susan Childs

A TASK FOR YOU

Take some examples of your own thoughts in this situation and see if you can identify any distortions or thinking errors. Look for alternative interpretations that are more supported by your actual experience.

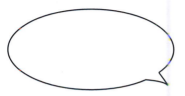

My alternative thought is ....

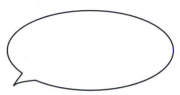

My alternative thought is

....

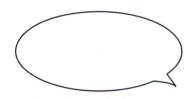

My alternative thought is

....

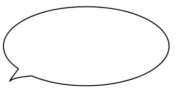

My alternative thought is

....

STRATEGIES FOR MANAGING PAIN AND INTIMACY

The first step is always to *discuss* the problem with your partner. This is the person who most needs to know your thoughts and fears in the situation in order to understand exactly how to respond to you.

You may need to explain that because sex was difficult on one occasion, it doesn't mean you don't ever want to try again. Partners often voice concerns about hurting the person with pain and you need to *take control and feed back how you are feeling.*

It is worth agreeing between you about all the different kinds of sexual activity you find pleasurable. Sometimes just lying beside each other and holding hands may be enough. You may need to explore ways of expressing affection and sexuality that are different from how they were before the pain problem.

> If you've been avoiding the subject for a while, you might find that you both notice your libido is low. This is particularly true if you have low mood, have low self-esteem and have made little opportunity for practice. However, don't despair – libido will increase with practice and confidence. All it takes is time, patience and experimentation. You might want to start with masturbation so that you can really explore what's good for you. This would be a good time to experiment with sex toys if you feel like it.

An important next step is to *make time.* Create an opportunity and prioritise activities that set a romantic scene.

> Engage all your senses: use scented candles, soft music and gentle touches, and feed each other chocolate or strawberries. If you like, watch an X-rated film.

The next step is *to define the goal* that you are aiming for on each occasion.

You don't need to assume that full intercourse and simultaneous orgasms are the only real expressions of proper sex. Take control and set pacing limits the same as you would for any other activity.

For example, you might suggest two or three minutes kissing while sitting on the sofa and then a rest before trying again.

When you want to progress you could take a warm bath or shower together and then try massage.

Speechmark Ⓢ Ⓟ This page may be photocopied for instructional use only © 2014 Keren Fisher and Susan Childs

EXPLORING AND FEEDING BACK YOUR RESPONSES

The technique known as 'sensate focus' is excellent for helping with communication about what you each find enjoyable. Each partner takes it in turn to be the giver and the receiver of a gentle massage.

The first sensate exercise is intended to avoid any direct genital stimulation, so there is no demand for 'being ready' or going too far or too fast.

As the person with pain, you take the receiver role first. You can lie in any comfortable position, using pillows, cushions or towels to support your back, neck and knees. Your partner uses baby oil or lotion and massages your arms, legs and upper body, back and front if you wish.

Your responsibility is to tell your partner what you feel. Use phrases like, 'That's very nice like that', or 'Do it a bit slower', or 'Do a bit more of this but a bit less of that', 'Try this area here'. Keep telling your partner what you like. Don't concern yourself with how your partner is feeling. Your responsibility is to be entirely selfish and focus on your own reactions. *The only goal at the moment is to learn what feels good and to communicate it.*

When you have had enough, swap roles. Get into a comfortable position to be the giver and massage your partner in a similar way, encouraging feedback about what he or she likes best.

Practise this exercise a few times to get really familiar with your preferences and those of your partner. Try short sessions, little and often, so that you don't get too tired or stiff, but remember, *pain does not mean harm.* You may have an increase in pain from overusing some muscles that aren't used to it, but this is *good* pain.

Actually, sexual stimulation itself is often a useful painkiller, as it is relaxing and it releases brain chemicals such as endorphins – feel-good substances – and oxytocin. This reduces anxiety and increases trust and bonding, not only between mothers and babies, but between partners too. These chemicals are known to help relieve pain.

Feel good

When you feel ready, you can be more adventurous and incorporate some direct genital stimulation if you wish. There still need be no demand for penetration. Mutual masturbation to climax can be the agreed goal. Keep telling each other what feels good.

Speechmark Ⓢ Ⓟ This page may be photocopied for instructional use only © 2014 Keren Fisher and Susan Childs

SOME SUGGESTED POSITIONS

When you both agree, you can try exploring new positions for intercourse.

As the person in pain you may be more comfortable lying on your back, with your legs well supported by pillows. Your partner can then approach you by kneeling so that you don't feel too crushed or restricted.

If it feels better for you, you could lie on your front so your partner can approach you from behind. Use pillows to support your chest and stomach so your back is in a comfortable position – not too extended.

Side to side is good if you don't like lying flat. Arrange your legs over each other, so you can stimulate each other as much as you want.

If you prefer, you could get on top with your knees either side of your partner's legs. This is good for back pain as it allows you to bend forward or backwards to achieve the most comfortable position.

You could also try sitting on a chair without arms but with a comfortable seat, with your partner in your lap, facing towards you – good for intimate cuddles and kissing.

Or you could sit on your partner's lap both facing in the same direction. This is good for both of you to have your hands free. You can take your partner's hands and demonstrate the stimulation you want – known as the 'hand riding' technique.

If you both agree, you could try oral sex.

If you want to use a vibrator or a similar aid, check that you both agree, so that neither can think it's because of some personal inadequacy or failure.

Invent your own experiments to see what suits you both.

There are only two rules you need to follow.

Rules	
1	Keep exploring and communicating what's good for you both
2	Remember to have *fun*

Speechmark P This page may be photocopied for instructional use only © 2014 Keren Fisher and Susan Childs

MAKING NEW RELATIONSHIPS

The concern some patients with pain have when thinking about meeting new people is how much to disclose about the limitations the pain problem imposes on their lives. On the one hand, they quite rightly believe that the pain does not define them, but on the other hand, they don't want to be seen as unsociable or standoffish because they don't participate in some of the others' favourite pastimes.

This is a dilemma that needs a plan and practice at putting it into operation.

Any new relationship, however meaningful or short-lived, may well start with you and your potential friends having a social pursuit in common. Choose the activity carefully so that it is not too physically demanding for you, and so it may be possible even on a bad pain day. For example, an activity such as a reading group where you need only say that you prefer to stand for some of the time may be more comfortable than a walking club where you might feel anxious about keeping up.

If you have learned to accept your pain and its limitations, you could consider joining a support group for people with similar problems, or starting one if that would be more convenient. You may want to direct the conversation a bit so that the meetings don't all end up focusing on complaints rather than coping strategies.

If you manage to meet a potential dating partner, you need all your assertiveness skills to communicate your problem without killing the relationship stone dead at the first hurdle.

You could decide to tell this person early on that you are very *interesting and creative* but you have something important to say. That way your story will be taken seriously and your partner can make a choice about how to respond. If he or she sticks around, you could both go to sessions in your pain management programme (*see* Section 17, 'Family and Friends') so that your partner is fully informed about your condition and what to expect from you.

You need to explain that sometimes the pain will make it difficult to communicate your needs clearly and that you might look as if you are signalling anger or distress when you don't mean to be.

Partners too need to be honest about their reactions to what they are taking on. They will not be able to *fix* you and they must accept that their role cannot expect to achieve this.

With confidence, good humour and good communication on both sides, valuable and fulfilling relationships can flourish.

Self-esteem and Chronic Pain

15

The experience of chronic pain often affects the way people feel about themselves, because it has such enormous effects on their lifestyles.

> People can start to define themselves by their pain and not by other aspects of their personalities.

Self-esteem can be considered as a sense of your value as a person. Although before your pain problem you might have felt quite competent to deal with life's challenges, chronic pain can make a big difference to your confidence about yourself. Your self-esteem may have become much more vulnerable to your mood and to your sense of achievement at any one time.

Where did your self-esteem come from in the first place? The answer is most likely from your early childhood experiences.

- **Good self-esteem**. If you are fortunate, you will have lived in a circle of people who believed everyone deserves to be listened to. You were congratulated for your achievements, and your weaknesses were acknowledged realistically. By interacting with people who reinforced your experience of competence and happiness, you developed a sense of good self-worth.
- **Low self-esteem**. On the other hand, you may have learned that you only achieved positive attention from the people who are important to you if you behave in certain ways (such as doing well in tests and obeying commands). This will leave you uncertain about your own judgement and fearful that others will criticise you. You are especially afraid of making mistakes in case people disapprove of you.

CORE BELIEFS

If you were bullied or abused by older people at home or at school, you may have developed a *core belief* about yourself that you are worthless and unlovable. This will then tend to form the filter through which you view later life experiences. Any small problem will seem to reinforce your low self-worth.

 Speechmark ⓟ This page may be photocopied for instructional use only © 2014 Keren Fisher and Susan Childs

SOME CHARACTERISTICS OF PEOPLE WITH LOW SELF-ESTEEM

People with low self-esteem do not believe they are entitled to love and respect. They will be sensitive to even mild criticism and will have little confidence in their own ability to meet the stresses in their lives. They will tend to see temporary problems as proof that they are incapable of leading the life they want. If you asked them to insert on a chart, they might fill it in as shown in this pie chart.

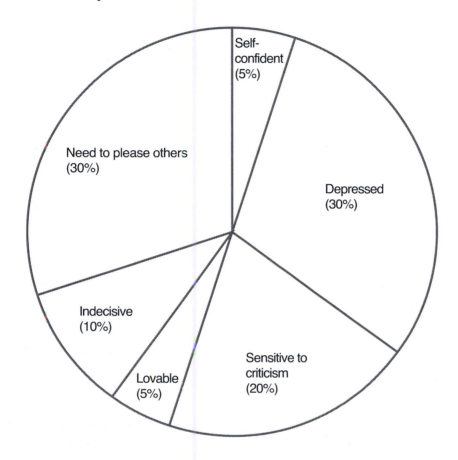

Their negative mental filter means that even well-intentioned comments from friends get caught up in a vicious circle. This can lead to avoidance of social interaction as a protection against feeling anxious and low.

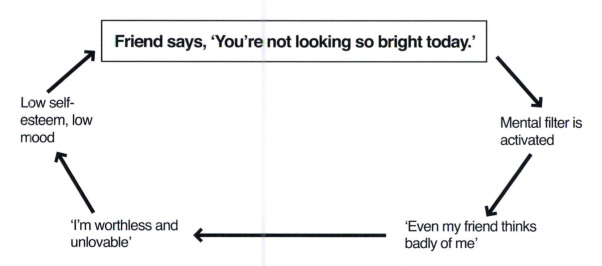

Speechmark ⑤ ℗ This page may be photocopied for instructional use only © 2014 Keren Fisher and Susan Childs

SOME CHARACTERISTICS OF PEOPLE WITH GOOD SELF-ESTEEM

People with good self-esteem will tend to rely on their *own ability* to solve problems but they do not feel guilty about asking for help if they need it. They will not waste time regretting the past or worrying about the future, and they do not allow their opinions to be swayed by others, unless it seems convenient. Their pie chart might look like the one shown here.

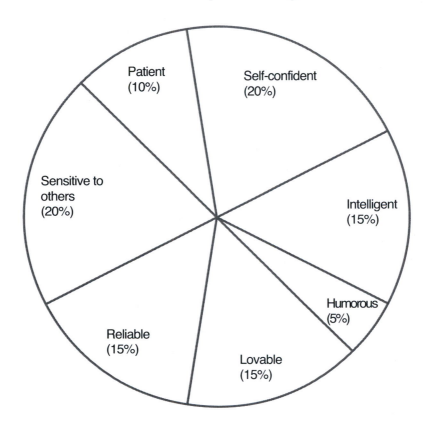

Their self-concept has developed from the experience of being spoken to and listened to respectfully. Their shortcomings are accepted without undue criticism. If they are challenged about their actions or opinions, they are able to defend themselves while paying attention to the alternative point of view.

People with good self-esteem tend to elicit these responses by offering others the same reactions. They are able to form supportive relationships.

> Maintaining good self-esteem involves interacting with other people who share your values. They behave in ways you agree are for the best, while allowing everyone's point of view to be respected.

Speechmark Ⓟ This page may be photocopied for instructional use only © 2014 Keren Fisher and Susan Childs

A TASK FOR YOU

Have you noticed any change in the way you feel about yourself since you have been dealing with the pain?

Any *good* things?   Any *bad* things?

_____   _____

_____   _____

_____   _____

_____   _____

Fill in the pie chart here with all the qualities you think make up the kind of person you are. Try to make the slices approximately the size of the proportion of each attribute. The total should add up to 100%.

If you want to measure your self-esteem, there's a questionnaire at www.queendom.com (scroll down to 'Attitude & Lifestyle tests …').

Speechmark Ⓟ This page may be photocopied for instructional use only © 2014 Keren Fisher and Susan Childs

DOES HAVING PAIN RATE AMONG THE CHARACTERISTICS THAT DEFINE PEOPLE?

It does not appear in either the 'low' self-esteem pie chart or the chart for the 'good' self-esteem example.

The features that are rated as important when evaluating people are to do with *higher* personality qualities rather than physical ones.

> Having pain or being physically attractive are not characteristics that are usually associated with the way we value people.
>
> *They need not form part of the way you feel about yourself.*

It seems that although pain might affect how we view ourselves, a lot of this can be linked to the way we think and feel. This in itself links us to a wider picture than just pain. We identified that self-esteem does not just come from ourselves but also from other people around us and we need regular contact with others and a larger life outside of the pain to maintain good levels of self-esteem.

This will involve making sure that your social contacts reinforce rather than reduce your sense of self-worth and this will naturally lead to examination of *your own mental filter.*

> Are you interpreting others' comments so that they appear to be criticisms? Is your core belief that you are worth less now you have pain?

Core beliefs might be perpetuated by self-talk. The things you tell yourself can keep your self-esteem low. The thought 'I am worth less now I have pain' is an interpretation. *It is not a fact.*

Core beliefs can be treated the same as any other thinking distortion. PUDDING thoughts (those that are Plausible, Unhelpful, Distorted, Demoralising, Involuntary, Negative and Groundless) fall into categories such as overgeneralising, mind reading, jumping to conclusions and labelling yourself inappropriately.

Examples of self-talk, which reduces self-esteem

- *'I don't have what it takes to manage my problems now.'*
- *'I can't achieve what I want until I find a cure for my pain.'*
- *'I am not the person I was any more.'*
- *'My friends will soon lose interest in me now I have this pain.'*

Can you identify your own self-talk that is keeping your self-esteem low?

Speechmark | P | This page may be photocopied for instructional use only © 2014 Keren Fisher and Susan Childs

A TASK FOR YOU

Fill in this table to challenge core beliefs and negative self-talk.

When I feel low, the things I say about myself are:	What is the evidence against these thoughts?	My alternative self-talk is:

Speechmark P This page may be photocopied for instructional use only © 2014 Keren Fisher and Susan Childs

IMPROVING SELF-ESTEEM

Challenging negative core beliefs about your worth as a person may seem like a difficult task but there are lots of other things you can do as well.

Some people value getting fit or socialising more in order to feel better about themselves.

- Join a gym or find an exercise class. Do what you can within your pain limits and gradually progress.
- Find things you *enjoy* doing and *do more of them*.
- Do something helpful for someone else.
- Think about what you can do to compensate for the things you are not good at.
- Pretend you are like a person you admire. Act the role until it becomes more natural for you to behave like that person.
- If you are good at something, show other people how you do it and accept their approval with a big smile.
- Remember to use self-talk that increases self-esteem. Use statements like:
  - ❫ I am quite good at … (e.g. listening to people when they need support)
  - ❫ I can usually … (e.g. cook nice meals for my family)
  - ❫ I feel good when I … (e.g. persevere with a task until I succeed).
- Congratulate yourself as you would your best friend for your achievements.

You did it!

Speechmark ⑤ Ⓟ This page may be photocopied for instructional use only © 2014 Keren Fisher and Susan Childs

A TASK FOR YOU

Fill in this table with information that will improve your self-esteem.

The things that reduce my self-esteem are:	My achievements are:	I can improve my self-esteem by:

Speechmark ⓟ This page may be photocopied for instructional use only © 2014 Keren Fisher and Susan Childs

The Role of Exercise in Chronic Pain

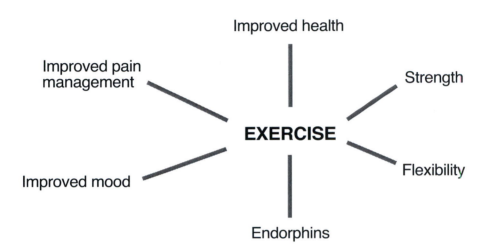

FIGURE 1 Exercise

People often rest more when they have pain. In the early stages after an injury this is probably helpful, but as time goes by it becomes a problem in itself and causes extra difficulties, secondary to the pain.

Rest reduces muscle strength and flexibility, joints become stiff and eventually even mild exercise is difficult because of lack of physical fitness. This in turn reduces self-esteem and increases depression, anxiety and frustration, as value-led goals get progressively more out of reach.

At first, the prospect of exercise after months or years of relative inactivity may seem a daunting prospect, but by starting with simple stretches, it's possible to encourage muscles to respond and recover without causing damage to the body.

Muscles will feel stiff after exercise but this is good pain, as opposed to bad pain that indicates new injury.

> *Good* pain equals muscle-training pain; *hurt* does not equal *harm*

Speechmark This page may be photocopied for instructional use only © 2014 Keren Fisher and Susan Childs

Exercise has a number of other benefits, such as:

- a general feeling of warmth and well-being
- the ability to carry out valued activities more easily
- improved sleep
- reduced risk of high blood pressure, heart disease, stroke and diabetes.

With all these advantages, it's easy to get motivated to exercise. However, remember:

You must take advice from your physiotherapist before you start.

Remember to begin with warm-up exercises, such as the few you can find outlined here, and only progress when your therapist shows you what to do next.

WARM-UP EXERCISES

Exercise target area	Method	How many?
Neck	Look straight ahead Pull your chin down to make a double chin Feel a stretch up the back of your neck	Hold for 5 seconds Repeat ×2
Shoulders	Keeping arms relaxed, circle both shoulders: ● forwards ● backwards	 ×5 ×5
Arms	Bring arms across in front of you to hug yourself Then bring arms back behind you	×5
	Swing arms up from your sides and straighten over your head and then back down again	×5
Pelvis	Place hands on hips and rotate pelvis: ● clockwise ● anticlockwise	 ×5 ×5
Knees	Bring knees up in front of you, as if marching on the spot Hold on for balance if necessary	Each leg ×5
	Hold onto the back of a chair Bend knees up behind you, lifting your heels towards your buttocks	Each leg ×5
Ankles and toes	In sitting or standing, alternately raise one heel off the ground and then the other	×5
	Alternately raise one foot off the ground and then the other	×5

TASK

 A TASK FOR YOU

Record how you got on with the exercises.

	Day 1	Day 2	Day 3	Day 4	Day 5	Day 6	Day 7
Number of minutes spent with these exercises							
What did you experience?							

Speechmark P This page may be photocopied for instructional use only © 2014 Keren Fisher and Susan Childs

IMPROVING YOUR POSTURE

People often develop bad posture habits without realising the strain this is adding to their muscles. Standing and sitting upright with the head well balanced on the neck and the weight evenly distributed through the pelvis, gives good posture. People generally have this instinctive position as small children but lose it over time.

Good posture can:
- reduce muscle tension
- improve balance
- allow better assertive communication
- increase self-confidence.

To achieve good posture in standing, think of yourself as a puppet being pulled upright by a string from the ceiling. This will encourage you to grow tall and straighten your spine. Open your chest to get your shoulders in line with your hips. Pull in your abdominal muscles a bit tight but not tense.

When sitting, remember to keep this position and use a cushion to support your lower back. This may need some practice, as your body will feel a bit strange if you have been a long time sitting hunched over a computer keyboard, or slumped on the sofa like most of us.

You can use a *mindfulness body scan* to check the alignment of your spine, so that you can notice the difference between the sensations of good and bad posture.

Put a sticker (or an app) on your mobile phone to remind you to check your posture whenever you look at it.

Simple Pilates exercises are very good for core strength to protect your back. See if you can find a course near you. The instructor should ask for any specific pains or injuries and advise you accordingly. *Ask your physiotherapist first before beginning Pilates.*

Family and Friends

This section is to help with running a session in which your family and friends are invited to participate so they can share the aims of the programme with you.

Your friend or relative has been attending the pain management programme and has learned about the importance of breaking into the chronic pain cycle (*see* Figure 1).

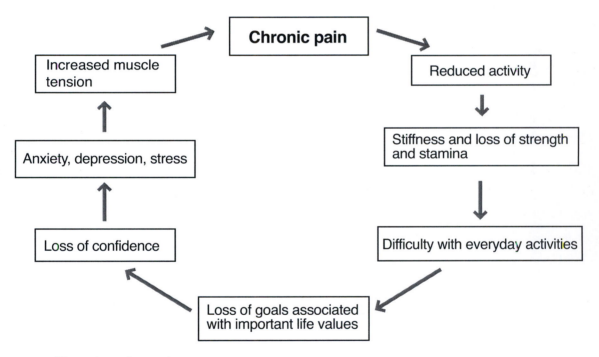

FIGURE 1 Chronic pain cycle

In order to reduce the influence of this ever-increasing circle on your lives, we have introduced topics on:

- pacing so as not to push into the pain and make it worse
- setting realistic goals in line with values such as improving relationships, work and personal growth
- looking at barriers that prevent progress

Speechmark P This page may be photocopied for instructional use only © 2014 Keren Fisher and Susan Childs

- identifying and challenging unhelpful thought processes and preventing thoughts being rules for inaction
- strategies for reducing the intensity of the painful sensations with relaxation and mindfulness techniques
- exercise in specific ways to rebuild strength and stamina.

As there is no longer a simple relationship between pain and injury as might have been the case in the acute pain stage, these strategies help to reduce the emotional impact of chronic pain on all your lives.

> A useful website can be found at www.bboyscience.com/moseley-pain

CHRONIC PAIN IS COMPLEX

> When pain has become chronic (persisting over time) it no longer relates to tissue damage.

In fact, emotions and memories are an intrinsic part of the pain experience and they have become more embedded with the pain in the time since its onset.

You may ask, 'Why haven't you diagnosed the cause of the pain so that you can direct the treatment at curing it?' This is an obvious question but unfortunately it doesn't have an equally straightforward answer. By the time pain has become chronic, many more pathways have been wound up into the network of nerve fibres that travel from the original site of the pain or injury, through the spinal cord and into the brain.

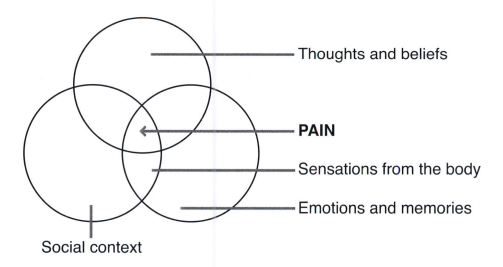

FIGURE 2 Complexity of chronic pain

Danger signals from the brain are now being sent *by mistake*, as there is no longer an acute injury.

The point of a pain management programme is not to cure the pain, as the original cause is probably no longer identifiable, but rather to reduce the influence of all the surrounding factors.

> Looking for a diagnosis has become part of the struggle that keeps people focused on their symptoms rather than their lives.

Lifestyle changes help the process of moving forward with important value-led activities rather than spending effort and resources trying to abolish or control the 'damage' messages. Pain will still be there but it will gradually take up a smaller proportion of life.

If you think a diagnosis is important, discuss with your person with pain how this would help the situation.

Speechmark ⓟ This page may be photocopied for instructional use only © 2014 Keren Fisher and Susan Childs

A TASK FOR YOU

Consider whether a diagnosis is important in pain management.

Has there been a diagnosis?	How did this affect how the family or friend managed the pain problem?	How did this affect how the person with pain responded to the family or friend?
Yes		
No		

Speechmark ⑤ Ⓟ This page may be photocopied for instructional use only © 2014 Keren Fisher and Susan Childs

PEOPLE VARY IN THEIR METHODS OF COMMUNICATING PAIN

Some pain patients may communicate in code, telling you that everything is fine when in fact they need you to notice the opposite. Other people might use various behaviours to signal pain, such as:

- guarding the painful part
- limping
- verbal pain complaints
- avoidance of previously valued activities
- grimacing or frowning.

These behaviours have several effects. Some might be used to reduce the pain but others are ways of communicating distress and eliciting help. They're not always easy to tell apart.

As onlookers, you might have a number of emotional reactions of your own to seeing your person suffering with pain and being unable to 'fix' it. You may feel frustrated and irritated or sad and concerned. Your responses might have unexpected effects.

- If you are *distant*, pain complaints reduce (according to research, pain ratings on a 0–10 scale reduce too) but the sufferer feels punished and tends to withdraw and to cope less well.
- If you are *sympathetic*, the behaviour that produced this response will increase – even more complaining or grimacing. This also reduces the self-esteem and self-confidence of the pain sufferer.

This tells us that attention to a particular behaviour will *strengthen or reinforce* it, so praise and encouragement for progress in important goals will be very helpful and will tend to focus everyone's efforts on life skills rather than on pain.

When progress is not going so well, you might notice cues indicating increasing pain, such as your person with pain getting slower, quieter or more stressed. You could then ask *if it's worth continuing with an activity and risking more pain* (it might be worthwhile occasionally) or if it would be better to take a break.

In this way, the pain sufferer feels understood and valued and attention is focused on coping rather than on unhelpful beliefs and emotions.

You may also notice that your person with pain feels more confident to express exactly what *you* need to do to be helpful in a situation. If this doesn't happen, you could ask for precise instructions rather than jumping in and risking doing the wrong thing.

> The best way to be helpful is by getting involved in using the strategies your friend or relative has learned to use.

Speechmark ⓈⓅ This page may be photocopied for instructional use only © 2014 Keren Fisher and Susan Childs

CHANGES YOU MAY HAVE NOTICED IN MANAGING COMMON PROBLEMS

What's new?

Problem noted by friend or family	Pain patient's previous response	Pain patient's response since programme	Family or friend's helpful contribution
I never know if I should help	Desperate for help but didn't ask	Asks for specific help required	Don't assume; ask what's required if it's not clear
My person with pain is often irritable	Got annoyed easily Felt helpless and unable	Explains why he or she feels irritable	Encourage relaxation, small goal achievement
Pain complaints fluctuate and are unpredictable	Expected to be understood	Honest report of good and bad days	Have fun on good days; encourage better pacing on bad days
Hard to get person with pain to join in our activities	Wanted to join in but too anxious about making pain worse	States assertively how much he or she can join in	Accommodate person's clearly stated limits
Person often very quiet and unsociable	Felt helpless and a burden	Explains that getting quiet is a cue that pain is increasing and that he or she needs to change activity or position or needs to practise relaxation	Respect the person's decision and not try to carry on with activity regardless (unless it is very important to continue and rest is planned for later)

TASK

    A TASK FOR YOU

Fill in your own problem list and discuss the solutions you would like to try out with the pain patient.

Problem noted by friend or family	Pain patient's previous response	Pain patient's response since programme	Family or friend's helpful contribution

Speechmark P This page may be photocopied for instructional use only © 2014 Keren Fisher and Susan Childs

Pain Management Programme Problem Pages

18

On the programme we have covered a number of ways in which problems that arise in your life and affect your pain can be addressed.

Be your own *Agony Aunt*.

Some of the techniques you may have encountered include:
1. recognition of distorted thoughts and challenges for them
2. acceptance of some discomfort
3. commitment to pursuing values-led goals
4. SMART (specific, measurable, achievable, relevant and time-based) goals
5. planning and pacing
6. mindfulness
7. defusion
8. relaxation and imagery
9. assertive communication
10. wise mind.

These techniques could be considered, alone or in combination, when you are confronted with troubles at home, at work or out in your social circle. You might also think of new solutions yourself that will get you where you want to be without increasing your stress levels and without sending more damage messages to your brain.

The following problem scenarios are examples of some of the issues other patients have raised. Choose the ones that are most relevant or interesting to you and see how many solutions you can come up with that would successfully and comfortably deal with the situation.

Remember:

everyone deserves to be listened to – that includes you.

You have been invited to your cousin's wedding in six weeks' time. You don't know him well, but other family members will be there whom you would like to meet. The wedding is 200 kilometres away – a longer journey than you can usually manage.

Your friend is a teacher who has recommended you for a post as a classroom assistant. You would really like to take the opportunity but you are afraid you won't have the stamina to deal with the children.

Your friend suggests you join a group going away for the weekend. You would really like to go but they will be camping and you need a proper bed.

You have met a new friend who would really like to develop a closer relationship with you and start dating. You are keen too, but you haven't yet explained to this person how your pain affects many areas of your life.

It's your turn to host the annual family party. Last time you made excuses and got out of it but you don't think you can avoid it this time. You feel really anxious about all the work involved.

Your child's class is going on a school trip. As your child has a disability, you need to accompany your child on the trip to help. You don't know how you will manage the long day.

You are just getting over a flare-up when your brother phones to say your mother is ill and she is asking for extra help.

Your partner suggests you try some new positions to liven up your sex life. You think they might be uncomfortable and cause you extra pain.

Speechmark ⓟ This page may be photocopied for instructional use only © 2014 Keren Fisher and Susan Childs

You usually cope with your flare-ups by using all the strategies you learned on your pain management programme, but this time you don't seem to be making any progress. Things seem to be getting worse rather than better.

Your children are growing up and you feel depressed and useless. One of them suggests you take a voluntary job, but you don't believe you're up to it and you are afraid it would make your pain worse.

Your best friend has moved a few kilometres away. There is no direct bus but it is an easy journey by bicycle. You haven't ridden a bike since the onset of your pain and you are unsure about making things worse.

Your sister has just had a baby and you have to be an important person at a ceremony. This will involve holding the baby for at least 20 minutes. This is more than you can usually manage.

Your friend asks you to take him to hospital for day surgery. This will involve driving in the morning rush hour, waiting around all day and then driving home in the evening rush hour. You usually avoid driving at these times.

Your daughter, with whom you have a difficult relationship, has now started relying on you for babysitting while she tries out relationships with men you consider unsuitable. You find the whole situation very stressful and the anxiety tends to make your pain hard to manage, but you believe you owe it to her to help her.

Your son's girlfriend has moved into your home with him. This creates extra shopping, cooking and housework. Your son has never been domesticated and his girlfriend wants to help but she works long hours and is often not available. You find the extra chores make you very tired.

Your boss tells you that the offices are reorganising and moving. You are in line for promotion but you will need to work longer hours and have a more difficult journey. You are pleased to have been offered a promotion but you are very unsure about managing more than what you are doing already.

You are having a bad pain day and you feel fed up and anxious. Your friend says that everyone has problems and that you make too much fuss. You don't want to fall out with this friend, but you find this sort of comment makes you feel even worse.

You have managed your pain reasonably well for many years but now you have been diagnosed with diabetes. Your GP tells you that you must make big changes to your lifestyle, which will affect your pain coping strategies, and that you must also exercise much more to lose weight.

It is nearly Christmas and you need to do your Christmas shopping. Your friend suggests you both go to a late-night shopping event where there will be drinks and special promotions in the shops. This sounds very nice but the town will be crowded and you have already had a long day.

You have heard of a new treatment for your pain problems but your GP will not refer you to try this new treatment without evidence that it will be effective. How can you persuade your GP and achieve the referral?

Speechmark P This page may be photocopied for instructional use only © 2014 Keren Fisher and Susan Childs

Coping with Your Flare-ups

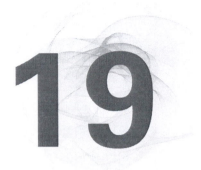

Flare-ups will happen. Long-term pain tends to fluctuate, sometimes because of something you have done but mostly because of factors outside your control.

A flare-up is a temporary, frustrating setback on your value-led journey.

A flare-up is *not*:
- the end of the road
- an indication that your work in learning all your coping strategies has been a waste of time
- an indication that you are back to square one and can never improve.

Flare-ups tend to occur when stressful events are happening, such as disagreements with family or friends or actual emergencies (e.g. illness or accidents). They may also happen in response to mood changes, such as depression over having to give up an unrealistic goal or the loss of an important activity (e.g. work).

It's useful to have a 'toolbox' pre-prepared, so that you don't have to waste energy finding your rescue remedies when you are already feeling sore and miserable.

Things to keep in your toolbox

- Instructions for gentle stretch exercises
- A relaxation CD or download
- A mindfulness CD or download
- Reminders to challenge negative thinking
- Pacing diary, for reminding you to cut back but to keep going
- Pleasant treats – chocolate, scented candle, magazines
- The telephone number of a valued friend
- Your own preferences: _____

_____

_____

_____

_____

You might also consider wearing simple clothes (although do get dressed rather than stay in your pyjamas) and eating simple meals that require little preparation.

Speechmark ℗ This page may be photocopied for instructional use only © 2014 Keren Fisher and Susan Childs

A TASK FOR YOU

You have probably already experienced flare-ups. It is helpful to think about what the risk factors were that led up to a flare-up. What was happening at the time?

What was happening?	Where were you?	Who was with you?	What sensations did you have?	What thoughts did you have?

TASK

   A TASK FOR YOU

When flare-ups happen it is important not to panic but rather to think of them as a PAPERCUT discomfort.

This is not as trivial as it sounds … look at it this way:

Prioritise – do what's important and leave the rest for another time
Accept some discomfort rather than struggling with it
Pace back, then gradually pace up again
Exercise more slowly for a while, but keep it up
Relax – revise your instructions and practise them
Commit yourself to continuing on your value-led journey
Unhook from 'disaster' thoughts – thoughts are not facts
Treat this as the temporary setback it is.

Fill in this form to remind you what to do during a flare-up.

Things I have tried that helped (do *more* of these)	Things I have tried that didn't help (do *fewer* of these)

Speechmark ⓟ This page may be photocopied for instructional use only © 2014 Keren Fisher and Susan Childs

Further Reading and Useful Resources

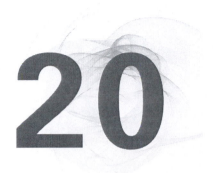

Butler D & Moseley L (2003) *Explain Pain,* Noigroup, Adelaide.

Cole F, Macdonald H, Carus C & Howden-Leach H (2005) *Overcoming Chronic Pain*, Robinson, London.

Dahl J, Wilson K, Luciano C & Hayes S (2005) *Acceptance and Commitment Therapy for Chronic Pain*, Context Press, Reno, Nevada.

Dryden W (1999) *How to Accept Yourself*, Sheldon Press, London.

Gardner-Nix J & Kabat-Zinn J (2009) *The Mindfulness Solution to Pain*, Raincoast Books, Oakland, California.

Greenberger D & Padesky C (1995) *Clinician's Guide to Mind Over Mood*, Guilford Press, New York.

Kabat-Zinn J (1996) *Full Catastrophe Living*, Piatkus, London.

Masters W, Johnson V & Kolodny R (1988) *Sex and Human Loving*, Little Brown, Boston.

Moseley L (2007) *Painful Yarns*, Noigroup, Adelaide.

Nicholas M, Molloy A, Tonkin L & Beeston L (2001) *Manage Your Pain*, ABC Books, Sydney.

Wells C & Nown G (1996) *The Pain Relief Handbook*, Vermillion Press, London.

Williams M & Penman D (2011) *Mindfulness: A Practical Guide to Finding Peace in a Frantic World*, Piatkus, London.

Willson R & Branch R (2006) *Cognitive Behavioural Therapy for Dummies*, John Wiley, Chichester.

WEBSITES

www.action-on-pain.co.uk
www.arthritiscare.org.uk
www.backcare.org.uk
www.breathworks-mindfulness.org.uk
www.britishpainsociety.org
www.expertpatients.co.uk
www.franticworld.com
www.getselfhelp.co.uk
www.painconcern.org.uk
www.painrelieffoundation.org.uk
www.queendom.com
www.youtube.com – search for Mindfulness Meditation Taster with Jon Kabat-Zinn
www.youtube.com – search for Lorimer Moseley Body in Mind – the Role of the Brain in Chronic Pain

 Speechmark P This page may be photocopied for instructional use only © 2014 Keren Fisher and Susan Childs

Index

Entries in **bold** refer to figures.